From the publisher:

Congratulations! Pregnancy and childbirth are certainly occasions for celebration. We are happy that you have chosen to let us be a part of this milestone in your life.

The Beauty of Creation is a wonderful book, replete with both inspiring stories and sound medical information. We encourage all expectant parents to use this as a guide to *supplement* the expertise of your obstetrician, midwife or other caregiver. While this book can make your journey even more rewarding than it already will be, it is not meant to replace the experience and knowledge of your caregiver.

Happy reading and congratulations again!

On the Cover: From left to right - Michelle Hendricks with her son Quinn; Elisa Roberson with her daughter Nandi; Lorinda Griffin with her son Shawyn; Zaakira Muhammad with her daughters Khadijah and Nefertari, as well as her son Seku.

Not pictured are Lorinda's son Kolby (ill with chickenpox at the time of the photo), Elisa's son Jair (not yet born at the time of the photo), and Michelle's son Blake (not yet born at the time of the photo).

The Beauty of Creation

Elisa Roberson
Lorinda Griffin
Michelle Hendricks
Zaakira Muhammad

with
Anne Graham, MD, FACOG, MBA
Perinatologist and Director of The Perinatal Center
West Palm Beach, Florida

NanKira Books

The Beauty of Creation: Inspiration for Pregnancy & Childbirth
by
Elisa Roberson, Lorinda Griffin, Michelle Hendricks & Zaakira Muhammad

Library of Congress Cataloging-in-Publication Data
The beauty of creation : inspiration for pregnancy and childbirth /
Elisa Roberson ... [et al].
p.   cm.
Includes index.
ISBN 0-9644932-3-3
1. Pregnancy–Popular works. 2. Childbirth–Popular works.
3. Motherhood–Popular works. 4. Obstetrics–Popular works.
5. Christian life.   I. Roberson, Elisa. 1967- .
RG525.B422 1998
618.2--dc21   98-40575
                                                   CIP

Illustrations by Tara Roberson

Special discounts apply for quantity orders of The Beauty of Creation. For fundraising orders, chapter reprints and other special sales, please contact NanKira Books at the address below.

NanKira Books is an imprint of KP, Inc.
Please address all correspondence to the following address:

NanKira Books
9506 Ridgeview Drive
Columbia, MD 21046

Contents

❧❧❧❧

Preface

xi

Dr. Anne Graham

❧❧

Introduction

1

❧❧

Chapter 1
Tell Me Something Good!

5

❧❧

Chapter 2
What They Don't Tell You
In Pregnancy Books

13

❧❧

Chapter 3
In the Beginning!

19

Surprise, I'm pregnant ✿ Welcome to your pregnancy

Journey from an egg to a baby ✿ Possible signs and symptoms

of pregnancy ✿ Wow, I'm really pregnant ✿ Your obstetrician

Expectations and reality ✿ Body Changes

❦❦

Chapter 4
You're A Mommy Now!

49

It moved! ✿ Heartbeat!

❦❦

Chapter 5
New Parent Preparation

61

New Parent Glossary ✿ The baby shower ✿ Preparing Your Baby's New Home ✿ Fathers

Are Expectant Too!

(New Parent Glossary appears on pages 61, 62, 70, 71, 87 & 90)

❦❦

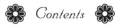 *Contents*

Chapter 6

Fathers Are Expectant Too!

81

What about me? ❀ Your role in labor and delivery ❀ After the big event

Chapter 7

Money & Your New Family

95

Chapter 8

Staying Fit

103

General considerations for prenatal exercise ❀ Pregnancy Workout Tips

High vs. low impact excercise

Chapter 9

The Wait Is Over, Here Comes Baby!

121

Don't forget the bag! ❀ What's in your bag? ❀ Reality sets in: memorable moments of

childbirth ❀ Childbirth! Labor and delivery ❀ Joy! Joy! Joy! ❀ Zaakira's natural childbirth

Midwives and midwifery ❀ Just be happy! ❀ Induced labor

Chapter 10

"Real Birth Experience? Having A
C-Section

155

A glance at a cesarean section ❀ VBAC (Vaginal Birth After Cesarean)

Chapter 11

Mommy's Milk...Does A Baby Good!

160

Colostrum ❀ More information please! ❀ Breastfeeding basics

❀ *Contents* ❀

Chapter 12

Hospital Eutopia

177

❦❦

Chapter 13

Tryin' Times, Cryin' Times

183

❦❦

Chapter 14

Complications of Pregnancy & Childbirth

189

❦❦

Chapter 15

High-Risk Pregnancy

by Dr. Anne Graham

199

❦❦

Epilogue

217

❦❦

Appendix A

Internet Directory To Pregnancy & Childbirth

Resources

219

❦❦

Appendix B

Prenatal Care & Nutrition

225

❦❦

Index

229

❦❦

My Pregnancy

239

❦❦

Preface

I am constantly amazed by the women I care for and the children that I help bring into this world. Though the miracle of birth occurs in that fraction of the time it takes for a new life to inhale and begin its journey, I am always unprepared for the feeling of awe that I experience at that moment. It is not that I am unprepared as a physician. Over the previous nine months I have watched the life develop. I have heard its heart beat so many times and kept rhythm with it. Through the technological wonder of ultrasound I have seen it move and swallow and wave in its cozy womb. But when I guide that sometimes molded head out, clear its nostrils and place this new life on a mother's belly to be welcomed into the arms of its family, I experience an overwhelming sense of awe.

Over the many years that I have spent helping to create families, bringing welcome children into loving arms, I have become even more appreciative of this great gift of love, of hope and boundless joy that envelopes all at that very moment. I had thought that with all the years spent caring for women and helping them at their birth, I would have become accustomed to the feeling. But this is not so. In fact, throughout the years I find that I have become even more emotionally involved. My patients have taught me much—about love, about strength, joy, hope, and how to deal with fear and sorrow. I have learned about being human, the strength of the soul and the natural resilience of a woman.

In the beginning, when I meet an expecting patient I must rejoice with her, but I know that this is just the beginning of a lifelong journey and the acceptance of

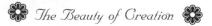

responsibility for another's life. Mine is for that period of pregnancy, but theirs is for the life of the child. I consider my patient, that mother, to be the watcher of her and her baby's well being. The times that I see her throughout her pregnancy are only minutes in the life of the fetus. I can interpret her symptoms and provide explanations for her concerns. She, however, must take the basic responsibility for care-giving. When she is lying awake at night, kicked by the tiny feet of the forming being, she will call me when things don't seem right. With the tools and technology I have available, and drawing on my years of experience, I will reassure both of us that her unborn child is happy.

In those times when tragedy arises, I share tears with my patients and try to provide explanations which may give hope. The strength of these women, the fathers and families that withstand their grief and in their despair wish to try again, reminds me constantly of the human spirit that renews and strengthens itself.

I am indeed in a blessed profession, being an obstetrician and perinatologist. I have a chance to see this wonderful divine gift and each time I do my spirit is uplifted by this miracle. On occasion, when the outcome is not perfect and I have to give bad news, I find myself drying both my patient's tears and my own. It is an incredible trust, one that I hold very dear and inviolate. Over the years, my patients have taught me much about love and hope and strength. I leave each encounter with a little bit more knowledge and a great deal more wonder at the beauty of creation.

Anne Graham, MD, FACOG, MBA

Perinatologist and Director of The Perinatal Center

West Palm Beach, Florida

Introduction

A friend of mine was in labor and going through some measure of pain, for obvious reasons, and delirium due to both pain and medication. At a point in time where things became rather intense in her labor, she declared loudly, "I hear voices! I hear voices! Can't you hear them?!" Needless to say, both her husband and mother, who were in the labor and delivery room with her, exchanged glances signaling to one another that the expectant mother had finally given over her sanity to the rigor of labor.

Her husband became very worried and while attempting to comfort her discovered something under the mounds of pillows resting behind his wife's head and back. It was the television speaker that was attached to the bed! So, his wife was in fact hearing voices, only they were not coming from her head, but rather from the television show that was on at the time.

❀❀❀❀❀❀❀

Congratulations! I assume that since you bought this book you are expecting, hoping to expect or know someone who is expecting a child. Get ready for the ride of a lifetime! When you think of a ride, you think exhilarating, fun, unpredictable and a plain old fantastic time. Pregnancy and childbirth are all of those.

I'm Elisa and "we" are the four women who have collaborated together with a wonderful editor and publisher to write this book. The story I just shared with you was one of a close personal friend of mine and it is an appropriate way, in its unexpected joy, to begin a book like this one.

Many books have been written about pregnancy and the process of giving birth, but our experiences as four mothers and friends led us to write something a little bit different. We are women who have been Blessed to participate in the most wonderful, miraculous and amazing experience a human being can be a part of, pregnancy and childbirth. We are more than sterile advice about what medications to avoid and when to ask for epidural. We are the sum total of 11 pregnancies and 9 births, from completely different life experiences and backgrounds.

The pregnancies and births were sometimes painful and filled with fear or worry, but in the end it is the beauty of it that lingers for a lifetime. The best advice that we can give is to Enjoy! Enjoy! Enjoy! You're more beautiful pregnant than you will ever be and this gift of creation is the greatest ever given. We hope we can help you to cherish it!

Chapter 1
Tell Me Something Good!

As you can probably tell by now, *The Beauty of Creation* is your pregnancy. It is about feeling wonderful about your pregnancy and preparing to give birth to those beautiful gifts that we call children.

Pregnancy can be a very memorable time in your life. This book was written to help you cherish each and every extraordinary moment of this time. Many people perceive pregnancy as memorable for negative reasons and often define pregnancy by trials and tribulation. Pregnancy is awe inspiring. Our perspective will be that of children and the birth experience as gifts.

Additionally, giving birth can be completely different from the sensationalized and crazed mothers in labor that we often see on television. While there are times that sensationalism and erratic behavior do occur, they are neither pregnancy's prevasive theme nor labor's defining moments.

God uniquely created our bodies to take on the magnificent responsibility of bearing children. The womb is sacred. To nurture, grow and develop another human being in your womb is a blessing from God. Our bodies were created so perfectly that during labor and delivery we just do what our bodies tell us to do. We have been given all of the tools necessary to make this experience successful, our job is to prepare for it.

The key to unlocking a positive pregnancy and childbirth

is preparation. Read! Read! Read! Study as though you were going into a final exam. Your pregnancy and childbirth are worth it.

However much we think we are in complete control of this experience, we are not. You couldn't stop a contraction if you tried. One woman going through her first experience with pregnancy and childbirth was in her 34th week. She had only had an hour's worth of minor back pain and one hour after this first episode of back pain, her child was born. The child, though premature, was fine.

The point is that your body will tell you when it's time, not the other way around. Your body will signal when it is time for the baby to come, that it is time for you to push, etc. And throughout the process you will be responding most to the signals your body gives you.

Of course, this process is not without trials, and sometimes tragedy. However, the experience of pregnancy and childbirth is so fantastically charged with good.

Elisa: I've always wanted to read a book about pregnancy that is positive and could leave me feeling goosepimply. When I first found out I was pregnant with my daughter, my first child, I went to the local bookstore that was supposed to carry virtually everything. I sat myself down in front of the pregnancy section, ready to read as much as I could and buy as many books as possible, but the titles I came across were negative. I had only known my baby for 2 or 3 days, but I already knew that this baby was a part of me and that everything I read, digested, did and said would not only affect my pregnancy, but also my child.

I was honestly distraught to find so many negative titles

and no positive. I believe in the miraculous nature of creation, the incredible nature of a perfect being formed with little or no conscious thought. Belief in a higher power or a God is a must because there is no way you can believe that Man alone could be responsible for making something as perfect as a child, time and time again.

Some of the happiest times of my life were during pregnancy. I felt the most whole and complete. Now I understand why they say that pregnant women glow. The bottom line is that it was just a lot of fun. I always had somebody there with me. Someone to play with, someone to talk to. I could rub my belly and know that there was someone there on the other side ready and willing to hear me and play along.

From the moment I learned of my pregnancy I already knew my children. Granted, I didn't know what they would look like or even what their names would be, but I knew the people they were. I was already proud of them like only a parent can be. I wanted all the best for them and even though I only knew them for a short time and hadn't even seen their faces, all the hopes, dreams, aspirations and worries of a parent were realities to me. I was already thinking about their first day of kindergarten or the first time they'd walk or graduation from college or even seeing my grandchildren. And this was just a couple of days after taking a home pregnancy test.

So bonding with your child before it arrives is really a joy and a blessing you shouldn't miss out on. Try to take advantage of this time when your child is solely dependent on you. Because, it seems like one day you're going to look back, it will seem like only a few moments have passed and they'll be teenagers or getting married themselves.

Zaakira: Parenting is an extremely multifarious process. It requires an immense amount of patience. It is also a venture that requires a tremendous amount of thought and planning. There exists no set of rules nor is there an instruction manual. Parenting is like a working document, there is always room for editing, growth and development. It's a process that is rewarding, yet one that requires a great deal of sacrifice. Afterall, when you are raising a child, you must make so many crucial decisions. Everything you do to help your child grow and develop eventually affects the child in one way or another.

Although I believe everyone comes to this earth with some mission to accomplish, it is a parent's job to cultivate and nourish a child to fulfill their predestined goals. Consequently, I am always enthralled with the prospect that I have such a wondrous opportunity to be an aviator for three passengers on the flight called LIFE.

Michelle: The entire process of pregnancy and childbirth is the greatest gift one can receive. It leaves me at a loss for words. I can't describe the love a mother has for her child, even while it is in the womb. It is completely amazing and like nothing else. Very early on your baby may give you hints about his or her personality. He may cry noisily or gently, nurse casually or vigorously. No one will ever know as well as the mother the unique individual she carried in her body for 9 months. And nothing in life will evoke the same tenderness, anxiety, fascination, and love as your baby.

Being a mother involves self sacrifice, my children were always first. Not only are you their provider and nurturer, you are their teacher as well. "Train up a child in the way he should go," (Proverbs 22:6). Children learn what they live and are a product of their evironment!

Most women are ready to deliver after 9 months of pregnancy, but I felt more comfortable pregnant. I felt a greater sense of control with regard to my child's safety. I had a greater ability to protect him and keep him safe in the womb versus out in the real world.

Pregnancy and childbirth represent the most important missions you will ever embark upon. Don't ever take one second for granted. Remember your purpose for being now is to love, support and nurture your child endlessly. My children bring me joy beyond compare. Of course, everyday isn't a bed of roses. However, you better believe that for every difficult day, you will have several rewarding ones. Enjoy!

The Heavenly Father chose to give me my son, Quinn, and a guardian angel is watching over him.

Lorinda: My belief about creation comes from the Holy Bible (from Genesis). God, who is awesome and all powerful, created the heavens, the earth, sun, moon and stars. And, man and woman were created in His image. He told man and woman to fill the earth with people. Having a baby is a gift to us from God.

Motherhood is a wonderful experience. If you ever experience any frustrations, the many joyous moments outweigh them. These moments are too numerous to count. Things like feeling your baby move in your womb; listening to the heartbeat; holding him or her for the first time; watching them grow "right before your eyes"; hearing those first words; little hands and arms reaching out to you to be held; the first scoots, crawls or steps; watching independence blossom as personalities take shape and the list goes on and on.

Being a mother means always praying for your children and teaching them of God's love so that they will love themselves and others. Being a mother is also sacrificing your needs when necessary, always nurturing and caring, continuously building your child's self-esteem and self-confidence, being a friend to your child, disciplining and loving unconditionally.

My children bring me joy. I think that they are wonderfully and uniquely different. Both are a little shy at first and will remain at a distance for a short while before they warm up to you. After that, they can be your best friend.

Elisa: The personalities of my children were definitely developed and defined in-utero. Like, my daughter would kick back really hard whenever I would touch her. She was strong-willed then and she's strong-willed now. In fact, we have video of her in the nursery when she was born. The nurses were picking her up to bathe her or something and she had grabbed the side of her bassinet. Keep in mind she's only hours old at this point. Once they gently pried her little fingers from the bar and went to pick her up again, she had latched on to the other side with the other hand.

My son was very playful and very mannerly, if that's a good word to use for a baby in-utero. It seems like he never tried to kick too hard or all the little curious things that a little gentleman would do, it seemed like he did those in the womb.

Being a mother, being a parent, being pregnant is just so joyous. I feel like the luckiest person alive and I really didn't want my pregnancy to end. And, just like most things in this life, pregnancy and childbirth are really what you make of them. If you want to be negative about it and think it's a bummer and walk around moping, guess what, it's probably going to be a bummer. But, if you focus on the blessing and the gift and all of the exhilarating moments that lie ahead of you, it will turn out to be a fabulously wonderful ride.

There are so few accomplishments in life that can never be taken away. Having carried my children and delivered them into this world is the greatest success story of my life.

I loved carrying them and being so close that they only needed me. What a power trip!

Chapter 2
What They Don't Tell You In Pregnancy Books

There is not a book in existence that can tell you everything you need to know going into a pregnancy and childbirth experience. Not all books will share this with you, however, and some give the impression that they have it all covered. Additionally, we feel that too many books are negative or indifferent about the wonders that a woman going through pregnancy and childbirth will experience. This was actually one of the reasons for writing this book.

We encourage you to read from as many sources as you can find, but we thought we would try and provide you with some of the types of information that you usually don't find in most books on pregnancy and childbirth.

Lorinda: From reading different books, I expected not to feel so great most of the time during pregnancy, however, the opposite was true with both pregnancies. The most valuable advice I got came from a friend just days before I was about to deliver. She knew that I was concerned because I was attempting to deliver vaginally after having had a c-section with my first child.

I was due any day, and I began to fumble through literature trying to find something that would tell me what to do and what to expect. My friend advised me that my body knew just what to do, just relax and work with it. She said to work with each contraction to push the baby through the birth canal and focus and envision the cervix opening that much more with each push.

Elisa: I was very discouraged by the fact that most books don't talk about just how miraculous pregnancy and childbirth are. When I first found out I was pregnant with my first child I ran to the bookstore and ended up sitting on the floor in the childbirth section and cried because all of the books were so negative or they were just very medical and sterile. I mean, there were titles that talked about pregnancy being the longest nine months of your life and this was actually part of the title! There were others that had phrases like "why didn't my mother tell me it would be like this" and "don't worry it will be over soon." I just cried and cried because I wanted to read a book about how this is a gift and such a Blessing. It's not something we can do by ourselves, it is something that the Creator is involved in and it is just so wonderful. I wanted to read joyful things about pregnancy and about childbirth and I just couldn't find them.

Michelle: I don't remember reading anything portraying pregnancy and childbirth in a positive light. I expected to feel horrible, sick and bloated. However, the contrary was true during my pregnancies. I didn't experience morning sickness with either pregnancy. I did find myself less energized the second time around, which could be due to having a child already or the fact that my current job is more demanding and requires a great deal of travel. I thoroughly enjoyed being pregnant. It is a beautiful and exciting experience.

Be your own judge. Don't let books or friends dictate

your feelings about pregnancy and childbirth! Your baby feels what you feel. Try to remain positive, happy, and upbeat as much as possible.

One tip: Warm prune juice is great for constipation. I didn't find that in any books.

Zaakira: I don't recall a time reading about how important it was for me, as a nursing mother, to rest while my baby was resting. I'm sure that it might have been mentioned in a few of the nursing books I read, but it wasn't stressed to the point where I took it to heart. I was so excited about the birth of our first child, I wanted to do everything "by the book." But, I found that I was becoming overwhelmed and exhausted when I tried to tend all of my regular household chores while my child was sleeping. However, when Khadijah would wake up from her nap, *she* was rejuvenated. Consequently, I had to tend to her needs. By the time I finished nursing and cleaning, I was completely exhausted. I was not scheduling time to do the things that I needed to do just for Zaakira.

As a result, I started feeling totally depleted. Whenever my husband, Hakim, wanted to share his day with me or just talk, I would find myself drifting off to sleep. This wasn't fair to me or my family. I had to create a schedule so that I could get everything that I needed to do completed, especially the things I wanted to do for myself which I would automatically give up to make sure that everything for my family was in order.

I soon realized that I needed that time for myself. I had to learn to schedule the necessary time for myself without feeling guilty. When I did begin to do little things for myself, I felt better, even if it was just taking an extended shower.

I noticed that when I took care of myself, I had more positive energy to share with my family. Now that I have three children, organization and planning are key elements to managing a household and career successfully. I am still not perfect, but I'm a lot closer to being an adept mother and homemaker.

Elisa: I don't think most books give you enough information about how really emotional pregnancy is; not just childbirth and having a baby, but how emotionally high and low you can become. I wasn't expecting to be on that much of a rollercoaster of highs and lows.

We hope that in reading our experiences in this book, you will gain more than the usual medical advice, but also a heart-warming, sometimes tearjerking, but always beautiful perspective on pregnancy and childbirth. And because the experience was so positive for us, forgive us if we also throw in a few stories about the joy you will experience when your baby has actually joined your family. Read and enjoy the beauty of creation.

Chapter 3
In The Beginning!

This may be the most exciting time of your life and is often filled with equal amounts of fear. You are beginning that glorious process of bringing a child into the world! But, you may ask, "How can I possibly go through 9 (really 10 because 40 weeks equals 10 months) months of pregnancy?" "Will I fulfill this role?" "Will I be up to the task?" "Will I be grown up enough myself to raise someone else?" "Will I love my children enough or 'right.'"

Or, you may be declaring to yourself loudly, "This is going to be great!" "I wonder what my child will look like!" "I don't know the first thing about raising a child!" "Where is that *handbook* that prepares you for everything?"

All of these and many more emotions are part of the natural gamut of emotional bliss and turmoil that may be experienced by expectant mothers. To be quite honest with you, no book can prepare you for what you are about to experience, despite the claims that many of them carry. However, what we hope to do is show you how this experience can be one of the most beautiful experiences of your life!

Surprise! I'm Pregnant

Elisa: With my first pregnancy, we had just gotten back from Africa and we knew that we wanted to try to conceive a couple of months after that. So, I came in from work and I had a home pregnancy test, because I was a little late and curious. I took the test into the bathroom and when I saw the result I started dancing around the house. There was no question that the red plus sign had appeared in the little window and I was pregnant. I danced and danced until my husband got home because I was so excited. Then I told him and we hugged and kissed and danced some more.

With my second pregnancy, since I conceived when my first child was 6 months and I was still full time breastfeeding, I didn't know that I was pregnant until I was almost 3 months pregnant. So, when I did find out I was in shock! I could not believe it! While I knew it was possible to conceive while breast-feeding, I just didn't think it was probable and I wasn't ready for that probability. So much for the books I had read and my doctor's confidence in breastfeeding.

Anyway, after the shock and slight panic, I was very excited because I had always said that I wanted to have children close together. I thought maybe 18 months apart and as it turns out they are 16 months apart, so it was perfect timing. But, I'm such a planner and organizer that I did feel a little out of control with this second pregnancy. However, on the flip side, I was happy that it happened the way that it did, because at that time I wasn't thinking far enough ahead to have my children 18 months apart had it not just happened by chance. I was also happy that it happened that way because sometimes with too much planning, things don't work out as well as you would like.

❀
WELCOME TO YOUR PREGNANCY!

Pregnancy is broken up into trimesters. Each is roughly 3 months long. Your pregnancy will generally last 280 days or 40 weeks, if you carry the baby to term (until your due date). If you do the math, that's almost 10 months, instead of the oft talked about 9 months of pregnancy. Your baby should be delivered between your 38th and 42nd week of pregnancy.

So, how do you calculate your due date. The most accurate way is by your ultrasound. They will calculate the age of the baby based on measurements taken of the amniotic sac, your uterus and the baby. Even with this, your due date is a guess, because there is no way to accurately predict the exact date you will go into labor and deliver; though you may have an aunt or grandmother who has been pretty darn accurate with family members.

When you see or hear you doctor refer to an EDD, she or he is referring to your estimated due date. To calculate, you must recall the date of the first day of your last period and add 7 days to that date. Then, with the date you get after this calculation, count back three months. There you have it! Your due date!

1st Trimester - It is good during your pregnancy, but especially during the 1st trimester, to abstain from smoking, drinking, other drugs, medication that hasn't been discussed with your doctor, and caffeine. You should make sure you take care of yourself because, as you go, so does baby. The first 6 weeks of pregnancy are critical to your baby's development since the major organs are forming and by the end of the third month your baby has a beating heart, arms, legs, beginnings of fingers and toes, reproductive organs, urinary and circulatory systems and a liver. Your baby gets to be as long as 3 inches during this time.

You should schedule your first prenatal visit and begin prenatal care, which includes adequate rest, exercise, nurtition and a positive attitude. Your doctor will probably write a prescription for prenatal vitamins and possibly iron and calcium supplements as well. You may experience fatigue and sleepiness, more frequent urination, tender nipples, slightly fuller breasts, indigestion, flatulance (farting), nausea and vomiting, constipation, food cravings, possibly some expansion of your waistline, and occasional headaches within these first three months. It's not as bad as it sounds! Everyone doesn't experience everything. You'll see that in the shared experiences of the mothers in this book.

❀

2nd Trimester - Your fourth month of pregnancy is the beginning of your 2nd trimester. Congratulations, you could begin to "show" somewhere around this time (fourth or fifth month). In other words, it will become outwardly noticeable that you are pregnant. Your frequency of urination may decrease and any morning sickness may abate.

You may notice that during your pregnancy you have some nasal congestion and nosebleeding. The nasal congestion isn't necessarily your allergies. Your body is going through tremendous hormonal changes. Your body's increased production of progesterone is partly responsible for your bloody noses and stuffiness. Progesterone helps build up the uterine lining to maintain the pregnancy and has a similar effect on the thickening of the tissue lining your nasal passages.

In the 2nd trimester, you may also notice that occasionally it is difficult for you to breath very deeply and you experience some breathlessness. Similarly, hormonal activity swells small blood vessels in the respiratory tract. Another contributing factor is your enlarging uterus and baby pushing internal organs aside, including your lungs. If you have occasional forgetfulness (or frequent) and confusion, don't get too frustrated. This is to be expected with a mom-to-be.

And again, bleeding gums may also appear because of increased hormonal activity. You also want to make sure that your bleeding nose and other symptoms aren't because of iron deficiency. Are you taking your prenatal vitamins and iron tablets?

Anywhere from 16-20 weeks you may be able to feel your baby move for the first time. It could range from a kick to a butterfly-like sensation to the feeling of gas bubbles. Don't panic if week 20 rolls around and you haven't felt baby kick yet. Each mother-to-be is different. Your baby will announce his or her presence soon enough.

Speaking of baby, by the sixth month, baby is as long as 13 inches and can weigh as much as $1^{1/2}$ pounds.

For mothers who may be worried, a slight vaginal discharge is normal during pregnancy (whitish discharge). And, occasionally a mom-to-be will have some spotting. Spotting is when spots of blood are visible in your panties or on toilet paper. This can happen when everything is progressing perfectly fine in your pregnancy. You'll still want to report it to your doctor and take note of the color. Bright red blood is a warning that something is wrong, as is heavy bleeding. Brownish to pink spotting could be perfectly normal. Your doctor will be able to reassure you.

❀

3rd Trimester - Wow! You're more than halfway there. Your 3rd trimester begins with your seventh month. At this time your baby is probably over 2 pounds and 15 to 16 inches long. You're getting there. You should really be able to feel your baby's movement now, though some babies are less active in the womb than others.

A little ankle swelling is not uncommon at this stage of your pregnancy. You may also have more of the heavy whitish discharge. As your insides get more crowded, flatulence and indigestion can increase. Don't be embarrassed, you have good reason for these side effects. You may experience some insomnia at this time as well. Braxton-Hicks contractions may be felt and don't feel clumsy if you do become more clumsy.

Around your eighth month your baby shifts into a position that it will stay in until born, with its head pointing down toward your vagina. Your baby is doing a great deal of growing now and you'll notice it as your uterus becomes larger.

If you haven't already noticed, talking, reading, music and loud noises get your baby's attention. Some babies are more excitable than others, but you should spend time communicating with your unborn child. Play soothing music and chances are that this same music will soothe the baby after it enters the world. Your baby is forming a little personality, or at least may be doing some of the things that you will notice outside of the womb. You can really see this best on your ultrasound visits.

Aside from some of the discomforts and symptoms of pregnancy you may have already been experiencing, you may have backache; leg cramps; discomfort in your backside and pelvic area because of the baby "dropping;" more frequent Braxton-Hicks contractions; a belly button that now protrudes if it didn't before you were pregnant; and more difficulty sleeping. Then again, you might not experience these things. Play it as you go.

You probably will have done this earlier in pregnancy, but to help with your sleeping comfort as your belly grows, try a "belly wedge." These are little door-stop like pillows that are sold in baby stores.

As you get closer to labor, you may feel the need to make yourself busy, building a playground for your child, putting a new wing on the nursery, rearranging the whole house, etc. Of course, this may be a slight exaggeration for some (and not for others). This is referred to as your "nesting" instinct. You are getting ready for your baby's arrival. Don't overdo it.

Hang in there! You're in the home stretch now. Labor and delivery are not far down the road. If your baby doesn't arrive on the exact day you predicted, don't worry, it's coming!

For a more detailed account of what you can expect throughout your pregnancy, continue reading this book. It's all there for you to absorb and use as both a reference tool and a comforting inspiration.

Good luck!

Lorinda: I was very happy when I found out about both my first and second pregnancies. I did my first pregnancy test at work. When it came out positive I was ecstatic, though I didn't say anything to my co-workers and surely not to my supervisor. So I waited until I got home to break the news to my husband!

Michelle: With my first pregnancy, I had no idea that I was pregnant. My husband was ready for children immediately (a honeymoon baby would have been just fine). However, I had many apprehensions due to the current condition of the world we live in.

Obviously, my husband had a very convincing story. I stopped using the birth control pills I was taking, figuring that we might start to try three months later. However, I became pregnant the first month that I discontinued the pill. The irony of the situation was this: in mid-December '93 my husband and I travelled to Florida to spend the Christmas holidays with my family. While at home I noticed an increase in weight. To put it bluntly, my hips were spreading. I started exercising and walking to combat the weight gain I was experiencing. Everyone was laughing at my sudden interest in physical activity, but I continued to work at it.

❀

CONCEPTION:
Most people are amazed to find out that the process of conception—including ovulation, the introduction of sperm into the vaginal canal, and the subsequent fertilization of the egg—can only occur within approximately a 9 day window each month. It's really amazing that as many women become pregnant as do (especially those who aren't trying).

However, even for women who aren't trying to become pregnant, the body is so profound that for many women it allows the increased stimulation of certain desires (sexual for example) during that narrow window of opportunity each month.

While I was at home in Florida I came down with a horrible cold and took every cold remedy known to man. My husband and I returned to our home. And, in early January my *husband* experienced what we would eventually recognize as "morning sickness" for two consecutive mornings. At the time we assumed he had contracted some type of stomach virus.

Later that month, my period was 2 days late. So, without my husband's knowledge, I purchased a home pregnancy test. I had to sneak around the house to perform the test. And to my surprise, the results were positive. I decided not to tell my husband until I went to my physician's office for a blood test. However, one day he returned from work having had a really bad day, so I wanted to lift his spirits and I told him I suspected I was pregnant. He was just as elated as I was.

The next day we went in for the blood test. It appeared to be the longest day in history while we waited for the results. When I phoned the office and the nurse told me the results were positive, I slammed the phone down and started screaming! My husband made a return call to the office to verify what I had just told him because he was in shock. We celebrated all night!

So as it turned out my husband's upset stomach was due to morning sickness, which I never experienced myself. My obstetrician told us that she had seen this behavior occur in a few instances. She feels it is due to the husband being so much in touch with his wife and the pregnancy that he experiences the symptoms. My husband also had cravings. He gained 26 pounds versus my 13.

With my second pregnancy, I again took the home pregnancy test. I was away on business at the time. I immediately phoned my husband from the hotel to share my glorious news. I was extremely apprehensive, given an earlier

THE JOURNEY FROM AN EGG TO A BABY!

❀ *On only one occasion per month, an egg is released from the female ovary into one of the fallopian tubes. During this time of month (ovulation), a series of changes are occurring within a woman's body. Progesterone is preparing the uterus to be able to maintain a pregnancy; the environment of the vagina, vaginal canal, uterus, etc., is changing from an environment generally acidic and inhospitable to sperm to one that is more basic and with more mucus to allow sperm to live longer within the female as they seek out an egg to fertilize. Under ideal conditions within the female, the life of the sperm can be as long as 5 days.*

After the release of the egg, it has a 12-24 hour life span during which it must be fertilized by the sperm or it will pass with the menstrual cycle. Thus, taking into consideration the life of the sperm and that of the egg, a woman tends to have an 8 to 10 day window each month during which pregnancy is possible.

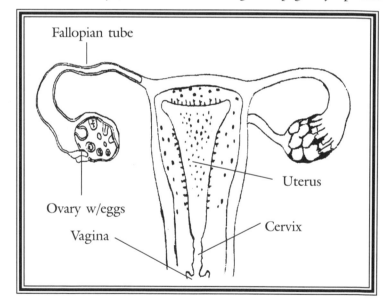

Once the egg is fertilized by the sperm, the newly fertilized egg travels the remaining path through the fallopian tube and implants into the uterine wall, which has been preparing for its arrival. Out of this ball of cells that was once an egg and a sperm, your baby and its placenta emerge to begin the process of growth within your body.

POSSIBLE SIGNS AND SYMPTOMS OF EARLY PREGNANCY

❀ *If you have a regular menstrual period that is a week or more late*

❀ *Breast swelling and nipple sensitivity*

❀ *Nausea and vomiting (morning sickness)*

❀ *Unusual tiredness*

❀ *More frequent urination*

❀ *Change (darkening) of color around the nipples*

❀ *Pigmented line forming, or becoming darker, from the navel to the pubic area*

❀ *Stronger than usual food cravings*

❀ *Positive home pregnancy test*

Other signs and symptoms recognizeable by your physician

❀ *Seeing embryo or sac with ultrasound*

❀ *Detecting a fetal heartbeat*

❀ *Uterus and cervix softening or cervical color changing*

❀ *Positive blood test*

❀ *Uterus and abdomen enlarging*

miscarriage. So, I searched for the best physician possible. This search led me to my current physician, Dr. Anne Graham, a perinatologist who normally takes patients by referral only. But, once I pleaded my case to the staff, they couldn't say no.

Zaakira: My husband and I were newlyweds when we learned that we were expecting our first child. We had only been married for 3 months. We had just experienced a beautiful and unforgettable wedding ceremony on the beach in Negril, Jamaica. We were both anxious to become parents. We loved each other so much that we wanted to create an extension of our love in the form of a child. We thought that we would truly be crystallized in the oneness of our Creator if we produced a child.

We both became extremely conscientious about our health. I wanted to be in the best condition possible. I paid careful attention to my body and I knew my approximate ovulation date. Consequently, after two months of praying, hoping and feeling disappointed when my cycle began consistently each month, I was ecstatic when I was one day late during our third month of trying so diligently to conceive.

I raced to get a home pregnancy test. When the sign in the little window of the test appeared positive, I was so grateful to the Creator for granting my wish. Then I carefully wrapped the pregnancy test in a plastic wrapper because I wanted my husband to see for himself that we had been blessed with a child.

I then immediately rushed to the nearest gift shop to purchase a bouquet of balloons for my husband. I selected three Mylar balloons, which proclaimed "It's A Boy!," "It's A Girl!" and "Congratulations!" I tied the balloon bouquet to a bottle of Sparkling Cider and sat the bottle directly in front of our door to surprise my husband when he arrived. When he finally figured out what was afoot, we shared a long embrace which I will never forget. We could not believe that we were about to embark upon the journey called "parenthood."

Elisa: When people say we're waiting for the right time or we'll know when the time is right for pregnancy, that really seems like a misnomer to me. In truth there's always one extra thing you can buy or one more promotion you're waiting for or another trip to have taken or another room to remodel. Unless it just happens or you make the decision to do it, in most cases there is no perfect time to start a family. There may be inopportune times and there may be less than perfect situations to bring a child into. However, in most cases, if you're waiting for the bomb to drop that's going to spell out in clear letters, in your alphabet soup, "it's time to have a baby," that may not happen.

However, I would recommend a) being in a loving marriage that's solid, b) being clearly defined with yourself and your God and c) a firm grasp on your own ideas and mores, and not being still in the flighty, exploratory phase of your life. It may sound judgemental, but it's kind of the closest to ideal that I can picture as far as being ready to have children.

So, no matter what your situation, I think two things are guaranteed. The first is that your child will change your situation and the second is that this change will more than likely be for the better.

There are some basic things that are good to know once you find out you are pregnant. First of all, are you really pregnant. Home pregnancy tests are not perfect and there are such things as false alarms. And, of course your level of excitement depends on a number of factors, so don't feel as though you should react a certain way to the news or feel guilty because you didn't react with a prescribed level of excitement.

There are many influencing factors on your reaction. For example, whether or not you were trying to get pregnant; whether or not you are married (we strongly recommend being in a good, loving marriage); whether or not you feel prepared, etc. The good news is that regardless of your particular situation, pregnancy and childbirth can still be a most wonderful and rewarding experience and an awesome responsibility.

Wow, I'm Really Pregnant?

It is ironic, but probably a balancing feature that the beauty of creation, pregnancy and childbirth, can be filled with fear, uncertainty and anxiety. This, however, is one of the completely natural aspects of becoming an expectant mother.

❀ **Miscarriage:** *We felt it was important to include information about miscarriage because so many women have them (about 30%) at one time or another and there is so little support or understanding for women who have miscarried. Chapter 14 talks more about miscarriage.*

Lorinda: In the beginning I was afraid of **miscarrying** and birth defects, but everything worked out fine. I gave birth to my children (no miscarriages) and they were healthy.

Michelle: After confirmation of my pregnancy, I went in

for my first examination. My experience proves that appropriate prenatal care is essential. Let me explain why.

I had been previously informed that I had fibroids. They had never caused me problems, so it was assumed that they would not during pregnancy. However, when I went in for my 6 week

> ❀ UTERINE FIBROIDS: *Fibroids, also called myomas, are benign (non-cancerous) growths that can appear inside or outside of the uterus. They occur in about 25% of women of reproductive age. They can be inocuous or cause problems such as heavy menstrual bleeding, pelvic pain or infertility. There are both surgical and non-surgical treatments available. We advice that you consult your physician if you have questions, as well as do your own research.*

exam, my uterus measured 12 weeks. This was due to the rapid growth of my fibroids.

Immediately, I was categorized as "high-risk." Luckily, I had complete and total confidence in my obstetrician and therefore continued under her care and watchful eye. Although she didn't inform me at the time, it was predicted that I would miscarry. At that point, I prayed to make it through the first trimester and so on. I can remember when I reached 28 weeks, my physician breathed a sigh of relief, because up until that point it had been touch and go. But, at 28 weeks I was pretty much home free!

All during my pregnancy, I feared miscarriage. Every time I used the bathroom, I was afraid I would see blood. However, as you get beyond the first trimester, these fears subside. I also became very protective of myself and fearful of the world around me. I became overly concerned about issues that I hadn't been before (i.e. politics, finances, rap music, education, family life, etc., etc., etc.). When driving I would stay away from the fast lanes and pull over if I saw cars swerving. I think I was driving my husband "bonkers!"

I remained positive at all times and avoided stress and unhappy situations. I played soothing classical/jazz music daily. Whatever I read, I read aloud. I ate healthier than I ever had in my life. I sincerely believe all of these things had an effect on the birth of my "miracle child."

A year and a baby boy later, I had my fibroids removed! My physician went in to remove 3 fibroids and removed 7. It still amazes me that my son survived. Quinn is truly a blessing from God.

Zaakira: Initially when you find out you're pregnant, it's an experience rippled with emotion. You realize that you and your husband have participated in creating a life. I was really excited about being pregnant, but I didn't contemplate it enough to be afraid. I really loved Hakim, my husband, and we were ready. We prayed for good health and I'll admit that I was concerned about my own health. But, I was really "gung ho!" I wanted to have a child that reflected Hakim and I .

I felt it would be an honor to guide one of God's creations through this journey called life. However, as the baby began to develop, there was a period during my last trimester when I felt fearful. I was so accustomed to having my child with me as I carried her that I did not want our special bond to break. We did everything together!

However, I knew that I would have to return to work eventually, and I was concerned about finding someone who would love, nurture and care for my child during her most formative years. At least while I was carrying her, I knew exactly where she was and I had an idea, due to the amount of activity she generated, of what she might be doing.

After she was born I decided to stay with her a little longer than I had originally intended. I was working at a private school which had an infant program. The director of the program allowed her to come to work with me and everything worked out fine! Even though I was working, Khadijah was in the same facility! We were still together in a sense. My prayers had been answered.

By the time of my second and third pregnancies, I thought I was a professional at harboring small vessels. Consequently, I did not have many concerns because I thought I knew what to expect. I later found out that each pregnancy was considerably different. My first pregnancy was great! All smooth sailing and no unexpected roadblocks. With my second pregnancy, I had an unexpected, fearful bout with a possible birth defect after Nefertari, our second daughter, was born. And with my third child, my husband was out of town. He did not get to the hospital until 6 minutes after my son, Seku, was born.

I noticed that I was extremely tense without my husband's presence. I had never lost my cool in the delivery room until I had to experience childbirth alone. Up until that point, I never realized that having the support of a loved one during the birth process is so crucial. However, even though the experiences were different, each delivery was a blessed event.

Elisa: My fears about pregnancy were miscarriage and not being competent as a parent. I had fears of not being a competent vessel, if you will, for a baby to exist within depending upon me for everything. I was really concerned, maybe overly so, about the things that I would eat, how much sleep I would get, the people that I would speak to, the movies I would see, the music I would listen to, or the tone of voice I would use. I wanted everything to be perfect for the baby and I knew everything I would do would affect the baby. It was a lot of responsibility. I wanted a "positive" pregnancy in every respect. I wanted to start nurturing and caring for and loving and being a real mommy to my baby the moment I found out I was pregnant.

Looking back on it, I really believe that all of those things mattered greatly. I wouldn't watch movies with a lot of violence or loud action, because I didn't want to scare the baby or let my moods adversely affect the baby. I knew and cherished the fact that everything that I did affected the baby. I wouldn't even argue with my husband because I didn't want to have any negative feelings toward him with the baby inside me. I didn't eat many of the things that I loved, like chocolate, because I wanted the best for the baby.

So, I guess a lot of my fears were based on things that I didn't want my unborn child exposed to. Fortunately, many of those things were within my control.

I also thought of things that I had never allowed myself to think of before. For example, am I a strong enough person to take care of myself and another person, forever if necessary? I knew that I could take care of myself, but never knew whether I was capable of taking care of more than me. The responsibility was sobering.

Your Obstetrician

Home pregnancy tests are great, but there is nothing like a visit to your physician to get the proper blood work done. And speaking of physicians, your choice of and relationship with your physician is an important part of beginning your pregnancy on the right foot.

Michelle: It is critical to have a physician you connect with, who is patient, and will empathize with your concerns. My physician was my first female doctor and I love

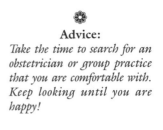

❀
Advice:
Take the time to search for an obstetrician or group practice that you are comfortable with. Keep looking until you are happy!

her and give her the utmost respect and credit for bringing my miracle child into the world. She watched me like a hawk. I was monitored very closely. In my opinion she definitely went above and beyond the call of duty. I often felt as though I were her only patient. My husband attended every office visit and she was very patient, addressing all of our questions and concerns.

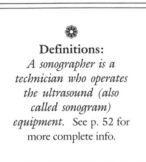

❀
Definitions:
A sonographer is a technician who operates the ultrasound (also called sonogram) equipment. See p. 52 for more complete info.

I never will forget the day Quinn, my first son, was born. It was the first visit my husband was unable to attend. I was having my biweekly ultrasound and testing. Apparently my "strip" wasn't satisfactory and my physician therefore requested another one. At the time, I really wasn't concerned because the sonographer (whom we had also bonded with, given the frequency of my ultrasounds) was very reassuring. However, after the second strip, I heard my doctor in the hallway say, in a raised voice, "Is this the second one?" At that point I was frightened.

She came into her office and sat with me. She tried to divert my attention by asking what we were going to name the child if it was a boy or girl. I only had a boy name because I felt as though I was having a boy the entire pregnancy. She smiled and then asked where Al (my husband) was. I responded. She very calmly said, "Give me his pager number and I'll have the nurse contact him and you go on over to the hospital to be monitored. And, if things look okay you'll go home and if there's any reason for concern, we'll evaluate the alternatives at that time." Her calmness made me calm, and instead of going to the hospital I went home to eat leftovers, get the mail, and my suitcase. This was four days before my birthday and there was a package on the porch from my mother, which included my birthday gifts and an outfit for the baby (I've always thought my mother was psychic).

Al came home and we went to the hospital together. I was monitored again and my physician arrived shortly thereafter. She came in and said, "How do you feel about delivering this evening?" I was in total shock. I think my husband nearly passed out. I said, "My mother isn't here yet."

I knew I had to have a c-section due to my risks and because my son was breech. My physician explained her reasoning, none of which I heard. And the next thing I knew, she was preparing me for surgery, as I was attempting to dial my mother and instruct my husband to get the cameras out of the car.

Al watched the whole procedure. My sight was blocked by a raised sheet. The surgery seemed to move relatively quickly. Fortunately, my anesthesiologist was a conversationalist, because my husband was so busy watching the surgery that he barely said anything to me. I didn't feel anything. If I had to describe that time period, I would say I felt as though there was a weight resting on my lower body.

There was a moment of silence...when they removed my son from my womb. It seemed like an eternity. Finally, I heard the wonderful cry of my newborn son!! I later learned (three years later) from my husband that there appeared to be a moment of panic when the physicians were delivering my son.

He told me that their faces showed fear and they began to work much faster.

While in the hospital recovering, my sonographer came to visit. We were in the office so often that we bonded with everyone. She informed me that on the evening my obstetrician delivered my son, she was not on call. But she knew I would be uncomfortable with someone else, because I made it very clear that I wanted her to deliver my child. She didn't want to add to my stress.

I also learned that she was due to go on vacation that weekend and expressed that there was no way she could have gone not knowing if my baby would make it through the week-end. I have always felt like I have a guardian angel watching over me.

All of this really reiterates the importance of a good obstetrician. Research and interview potential candidates. Make this decision one of the utmost importance.

Elisa: I think that for me, it was easiest to make a decision about who to use as an obstetrician, because Michelle had used her and trusted her. And I trust Michelle's judgement and respect her views as a mother. So it was easy to choose an obstetrician. I liked her and valued her role, but it was hard to bridge a friendship or camaraderie that you have to have to go through such an awesome experience together. It seems that you would want your best friend in there with you pulling for you and that's the kind of feeling I think most people would want to have with their obstetrician. I didn't particularly have that feeling with my obstetrician at first, though she was a great doctor. I didn't feel like we were best

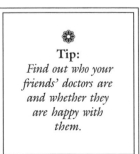

❀
Tip:
Find out who your friends' doctors are and whether they are happy with them.

buddies or anything.

However, after having the experience of fighting so hard in labor trying not to have a c-section and seeing the kind of person my obstetrician was, I gained so much more trust and respect for her. She was truly "on my side." She sat on the bed with me most of the day for about 7 hours and would only leave for a couple of minutes at a time. She coached me through contractions and things like that, and I know from talking to other mothers that this is not the kind of thing most obstetricians do.

The other thing is that she was patient and didn't give up on me, even when things seemed bleak. She seemed to sense and respect my fears and she didn't just blow them off trying to get home for dinner, or whatever. She really took pride in what she did and knew how valuable she was. She went above and beyond the call of duty, so to speak.

Lorinda: When my husband and I decided we wanted to have a child, we had been married for 4 years. My form of birth control had been the pill. When not using the pill, my period was irregular and I felt that I would have problems conceiving. My cousin, who had problems conceiving, had switched to another obstetrician. Soon afterwards she became pregnant.

When I heard her story, I called to get the name of her doctor. I really liked the doctor and felt confident I made the right selection. I did actually have to take a medication to regulate my period.

We were living in Virginia when my first son was born and he was delivered by c-section. While I was pregnant with my second child, we moved to Pennsylvania and I was again searching for a doctor who would give me a repeat c-section. A friend suggested a medical office where 3 women practiced.

During my first visit, I was impressed with the office staff and their efficiency. When I met with my OB-GYN, I told her I wanted another c-section delivery. She adamantly insisted that they only perform a c-section if it was absolutely necessary. There I was thinking that just because I wanted a repeat c-section I would be granted one. After that visit, I began searching for another OB-GYN (one who would give me a c-section), but instinctively I felt that this practice was one of the best around. So I decided to stay with them and thought to myself that I would probably deliver by c-section anyway.

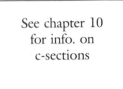

See chapter 10 for info. on c-sections

As my time neared and my visits became more frequent, I would now and then bring up the topic of a c-section delivery. My obstetrician, sensing that I was a little nervous, would gently encourage me not to be afraid of delivering vaginally. A vaginal delivery is what I had and things worked out fine.

Zaakira: I was referred to my obstetrician by a very good friend. She had been under his care since she had taken her first breath of air. He had delivered her safely to her mother as a baby and then she went to him for her gynecological visits. She spoke highly of him and I trusted her judgement.

I truly loved my doctor because he was extremely patient and always calm. Even in the delivery room, he maintained a level of calm that allowed me to remain calm as well. He also respected my wishes for natural deliveries. Whenever possible, he tried to explain to me what was going on at all times throughout my entire pregnancy. He also made sure that I went to classes on the process of childbirth.

His philosophy was simple. He believed that the more you became involved in the process of childbirth, the better you would understand your body and how it works. As a result, I felt extremely confident during all of my labors and deliveries.

Expectations & Reality

Elisa: I know every pregnancy is very, very different, as is every woman, but for me pregnancy was not as difficult as I thought it was going to be. I expected it to be harder work and, while it was very taxing physically and emotionally, I thought it was going to disrupt things more than it did. I thought it would throw life as I knew it for some kind of crazy loop.

Personally, it was a wonderful time of my life. It was not nearly as bad as I expected it to be. Now, it is not to say that this is going to be the case for everyone, because I know that there are circumstances where people have a rough, rough time. However, when I was getting ready to turn 39 weeks with my first child, I was sad and I cried because I didn't want it to be over. It was just that wonderful and such a joyous experience that I just didn't want it to be over. I wanted it to continue. I was so connected with my baby. We were so close, feeling every kick and wiggle. My baby needed me and I needed it.

Lorinda: I expected morning sickness and I was afraid of feeling queasy all of the time. I was afraid of not being able to return to my pre-pregnancy weight.

Michelle: I truly believe pregnant women have a glow. You're as beautiful pregnant as you will ever be. Don't waist a lot of time worrying about the weight you will gain as a pregnant woman. You'll have ample time to get it off. Enjoy eating.

My first pregnancy, although risky, was most enjoyable. No morning sickness, no cravings, none of the typical things you read about. I did have a bout with

> ❀ **Weight:** *Women gain various amounts of weight during pregnancy, and despite terms like "normal," weight gain depends on the individual. However, some women gain between 25 and 35 pounds during the course of their pregnancy. The best reference is that coming from your own obstetrician on your weight gain and the health of the baby.*

constipation, which warm prune juice relieved. I expected a lot of movement and my baby's movement was limited, again due to fibroids. People would often ask me, "Is this baby moving a lot?" How the heck was I supposed to know what a lot was?

Actually, I wasn't ready to deliver when I had to. I wanted to savor the moments a while longer.

My second pregnancy was a little different. I gained a lot of weight initially and spread rather fast. I craved McDonalds the first couple of months (I normally never eat fast food). I also craved iced tea and coffee. I was a lot more emotional, especially towards the end. I cried very easily. My energy level was minimal. I don't know whether to attribute this to keeping up with a three-year-old, or my age. Who really knows? And, the second time, I was ready to have the baby.

Lorinda: I didn't have morning sickness or anything. In fact, I felt great for most of both pregnancies. Then, there were the cravings. Everyone's stereotype about pregnant women involves their wild food cravings. With my first child I only had cravings for fried fish and cranberry juice. With my second pregnancy, I didn't have cravings.

Zaakira: I was waiting for the cravings, like ice-cream and pickles, but they didn't come. With my first pregnancy, I was extremely emotional however. I would say that my

---

❀ **Food Cravings:** *These peculiarities of pregnancy tend not to be random so much as the body's amazing way of obtaining the nutrients that your growing child needs. Your cravings often satisfy nutritional needs for either you or the baby, usually both. This is illustrative of not only the beauty of creation, but also the amazing precision and potential of the female body during pregnancy. However, don't get carried away and use this as an excuse to eat gallon buckets of ice cream. Neither you nor the baby need that.*

---

emotions were heightened. I analyzed everything that people said and did a lot of crying. My sensitivity level was heightened immensely!

Some days were more difficult than others, but it was all exhilarating. I loved every minute of each of my 3 pregnancies. I'm truly grateful to have been blessed to stand in line thrice for the ride called "Motherhood." Even though it was a rollercoaster ride of emotional highs and lows, it was the most miraculous experience.

Elisa: Everything was so intense emotionally during my pregnancies. Highs, and especially lows, might be bad ways to describe the experience, but it was just *intense.*

Body Changes

Zaakira: Of course, I had breast changes when I became pregnant. They were tender and I don't know if they looked bigger, because I've always had huge breasts, but what I could tell was that they felt differently.

My stomach color changed tremendously. It became very dark, almost black. My hair grew a lot as well and my nails

> ✿ **Skin Pigmentation:**
> *Some women notice changes in skin color during pregnancy. The typical changes are a darkening of the areolas around the nipples and the line (sometimes not noticed before pregnancy) that runs down the center of the stomach, called the linea nigra. Some African American women may have a more noticeable darkening of these areas, as well as in such places as around the neck. These increases in pigment tend to fade after delivery.*

grew. I think it was because I was taking in a lot of extra nutrients and eating more. But I don't know if that was really the reason why. People tell you that you have a certain look, a "glow," and I got that complement all of the time. Now whether or not it was true I have no idea. They could have been trying to make me feel better, but I was hoping they were being truthful.

Now I don't know if my nose spread at all, I guess you would have to ask my husband. I don't think so though. My pregnancies never really affected my face. I never had a big face or anything. I really just experienced a change in my hips and waist.

Michelle: I didn't experience a lot of the typical body changes during pregnancy, but what I did have were moles. Each pregnancy I get more and more moles. My grandmother had a lot of moles on her neck, so I don't know if it is just age or heredity. But with each pregnancy I get more and more moles.

Some of them disappear after the pregnancy and then others don't.

My neck doesn't get dark, nor does my nose spread. None of those typical things. But, I did have one hair that would come out of my chin and after my first child there were about 3 and then after my second child there were 5 or 6. With neither pregnancy did I gain stretch marks.

With my second pregnancy, however, I did get a couple of varicose veins in the thigh. And, my feet grew. I'm normally a size 9 shoe and during my pregnancy with Quinn I went up to about a 9$^{1/2}$. When I was pregnant with Blake I had to buy a couple of size 10 shoes. Now I wear a 9$^{1/2}$.

Elisa: My hair grew like wildfire! The first pregnancy I stopped cutting it and just started braiding it. It grew down beyond my shoulders in the course of those few months and I had to keep getting it braided every 3 weeks because it was growing so fast. And my nails just grew as quick as the wind.

With my second pregnancy my hair grew fast, but not as fast as with the first pregnancy and my nails hardly grew at all. Maybe it's a boy and girl thing, since I have a boy and a girl. Or it could be that my nails were just chipping off so fast because I had a one-year-old at home for my second pregnancy.

Everything also spread. My nose spread, my butt spread. It was just like a big spread. And my feet got bigger during pregnancy too. They did swell, but they also grew about half a size. I used to wear a 7$^{1/2}$ and now I wear an 8.

OTHER CHANGES YOU MIGHT SEE IN YOUR BODY:

❀ **CARDIOVASCULAR CHANGES:** *During the course of pregnancy it may be normal for a woman to experience an increase in heart rate. It can be as much as 10-20 beats above normal. The normal heart rate is, on average, around 70 beats per minute.*

Also, the amount of blood circulating through a woman's body changes drastically during pregnancy. Blood volume can increase by as much as 50%.

❀ **URINATION:** *Because the volume of blood in circulation increases during pregnancy, the kidneys have to filter as much as 50% more blood as well. As a result, urine production is increased. Additionally, kidney activity tends to increase when a person is laying down, which accounts for the increased frequency of urination pregnant women often experience while trying to sleep.*

❀ **DIGESTIVE SYSTEM:** *As your pregnancy moves forward and your baby begins to grow larger within your womb, more space is needed for your uterus, but not much more space is made within your body. As a result, your body improvises in its usually efficient manner and allows your organs to be pushed aside by your uterus. This may cause pressure on your rectum and large intestine, which is partly responsible for constipation some experience.*

❀ **DIGESTIVE SYSTEM CONT...** *Heartburn and belching also tend to be an untoward side effect of being pregnant. The lower esophageal sphincter (the circular muscle that surrounds the passage from your stomach to your throat and is usually tight to prevent the backward flow of food), tends to relax more and allow the stomach contents to flow back into the esophagus. Food also remains in the stomach longer, further contributing.*

THERE IS MORE ON THE NEXT PAGE, BUT BEFORE YOU MOVE ON, DON'T BECOME WORRIED. THESE THINGS ARE NORMAL AND WOMEN HAVE HANDLED THEM WITH LITTLE DISRUPTION FOR MILLENNIA! AND, NOT ALL WOMEN ARE AFFECTED. YOU'LL HAVE WONDERFUL STORIES TO TELL.

✿ **RESPIRATORY SYSTEM:** *Your growing baby and its enlarging home (your uterus) also tend to be partially responsible for affecting breathing. Breathing may become slightly more labored during pregnancy.*

✿ **HORMONES:** *During pregnancy, your body is preparing itself for one of the most miraculous events on earth. Consequently, almost all of your body's hormones are undergoing some sort of change. This increased hormonal activity often plays a role not only in mood swings, but also in many of the body changes discussed thus far.*

Progesterone is a hormone that causes the lining of the uterus to thicken, which is necessary for pregnancy to occur. This hormone also affects the way the lungs function during pregnancy and can account for the stuffy nose and feeling of congestion that some pregnant women experience.

Additionally, progesterone slows the muscular contractions that automatically occur in the intestine to push food along, which affects constipation.

The darkening of the skin and other pigmentation changes are influenced by a hormone produced by the placenta.

Mood swings are often hormone induced as well.

Breast swelling and nipple tenderness are often caused by increased levels of both estrogen and progesterone.

A wonderful array of changes are constantly occuring within the body of a pregnant woman. When this is understood in all of its complex glory, it is much easier to cope with. It requires understanding and, as the song goes, those around the mother-to-be should, "try a little tenderness."

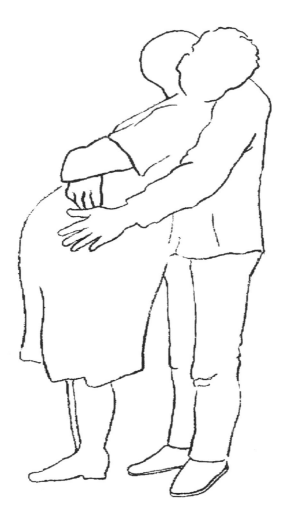

Chapter 4
You're a Mommy Now!

Welcome to the club. Motherhood doesn't start when you have a baby in your arms, it has already started with the one in your womb.

Zaakira: The time of my first sonogram was very memorable. I had never known anyone who was expecting, so seeing the baby in the womb was mind-boggling. I was so touched and I went immediately to the store and got a frame to put the picture in and show my husband.

It's so amazing, with technology being what it is today, that a parent can actually view the intricacies of their child's internal organs before actually seeing what their child's outward appearance is. I think seeing my child's heart beat and viewing all of the organs, which were visible on the monitor during my sonograms, really allowed me to understand the sheer miracle of life and the beauty of creation.

Michelle: My first ultrasound was a memorable experience, knowing that there was an actual little person developing and growing inside of me was phenomenal. My husband and I had done a lot of reading and we became pretty good at reading the ultrasounds. We were having them done so frequently, we couldn't help but become experts.

With our first son, we (or I should say "I") didn't want to know the sex, although I felt I was having a boy with both pregnancies (woman's intuition). The sonographer would look at our sonogram with caution, because Al was pretty astute at determining the sex. With our second pregnancy and a series of ultrasounds, we were pros. I gave in and let my husband find out the sex. Another boy!

Lorinda: It was hard to believe that there was a baby there. That little spot on the screen was my baby.

Elisa: When we first saw the ultrasound I thought that they were wonderful and it was so touching to see Nandi for the first time. With Jair I thought we were pros, so I was trying to find all of

❋ **Ultrasounds and sonograms:**

Ultrasounds, also known as sonograms, are a safe, painless and very common way to get a good approximation of the date you conceived, whether the growth of your developing baby is normal and a lot of other helpful information.

With ultrasound scanning an imaging device is connected to a monitor. The device is placed on the pregnant mother's belly and used to produce high quality images of what's going on in the womb, real time!

Nowdays, with a normal pregnancy, at least one ultrasound is performed to give the doctor helpful information about your baby and allow anxious parents to get a glimpse of the baby. That's right new parents, you can see your baby moving around in mommy's belly. You can even see and hear your baby's hearbeat as early as 12 weeks into your pregnancy.

Usually when ultrasounds are performed, the pregnant mother is asked to fill her bladder by drinking lots of fluids, as this allows for a clearer view of the uterus. This, however, is not necessary when the alternative imaging device, a vaginal probe, is used.

The vaginal probe may be used in very early pregnancy and under other conditions which favor this type of imaging. Your physician will make those decisions and be able to tell you why.

his parts.

When we first started getting ultrasounds I couldn't see the monitor as well as my husband, so I would read his expression to see if anything was visible or if the right parts of the body were in place. But, since my husband is not a very expressive person, it was very difficult to read his emotions, so I would get worried until the technician would say something about what could be seen.

With Nandi at about 28 weeks, we were feeling all around and she was very active. Her foot happened to be pressed up against my belly and the technician was tickling her foot and she would kick in response. We were able to see that on the sonogram.

Jair was so active that we couldn't get a good profile picture because he kept moving around so much. The only thing we were able to really see was that he was a boy because his legs were always spread.

It Moved!

Lorinda: The first movement I felt was a little flutter, but thrilling nonetheless. The baby mainly moved whenever I was hungry and the movements felt like it was stretching. As I grew larger over the 9 months, the movements felt more like thumps.

Elisa: The first time I felt Nandi kick was when I was in the bathtub, 16 or maybe 17 weeks pregnant. All of a sudden it felt like a butterfly flew through my stomach and I screamed out. My husband was on the phone with his mother and he came running up the stairs because he thought something was wrong. He was saying, "What...what's the matter, what's wrong!" and I said, "I felt it! I really did, I swear I felt it!" I was laying there rubbing my stomach and my husband forgot he was on the phone with his mother. Anyway, after that I took a bath everyday for about a week trying to get her to move again.

With Jair, Nandi would kiss my belly and rub it and Jair would move in response to her. She talked to him and he moved wherever and whenever she talked.

Michelle: The initial movements of my first child were infrequent and faint. Because I had never been pregnant before, I didn't know what to expect. When my baby first moved I didn't realize it was the baby, I thought I was just feeling gas bubbles, until my obstetrician clarified it for me.

It used to irritate me when people would ask if my baby was really moving a lot. Firstly, I didn't have anything by which to gauge "a lot." Secondly, due to my fibroids, movement was at best somewhat limited. I do remember early one morning, my husband was watching my belly

> ❀
>
> **Fetal Movement:**
> *The mother will usually always feel her developing baby moving in her womb before the doctor does. And, these movements are usually always different. From butterfly-like flutters, to kicks, to first baby movements mistaken for gas bubbles, each mother will be able to identify their unique baby's movements in the womb, usually anywhere from 16-20 weeks. But, if week 20 rolls around and you haven't felt anything yet, don't panic. Chances are, if you're seeing your doctor for your pre-natal care and keeping yourself healthy, everything will be fine.*

and he swore Quinn did a flip. He was so excited and intrigued!

When I was pregnant with our second son, I quickly learned what a lot of movement meant. He was most active between 9:00pm and midnight. He would move when Al and Quinn would talk to my belly, or when our dog barked.

Zaakira: All of my children have different personalities. It was evident in the womb and still today. My oldest daughter, Khadijah, was a very calm baby in the womb. She appeared to only move during the evening hours. However, she was intrigued by instrumental music.

I remember during my eighth month of pregnancy, I was invited by a friend of mine to a ballet recital. The ballet performers danced to live music. I was sitting with a friend and we both noticed that whenever the pianist had a solo, the baby would move so vigorously that you could literally see my jacket moving because she was so excited. Needless to say, Khadijah has an extremely calm, low keyed personality, yet she is very fond of ballet and many different genres of music.

Nefertari, my younger daughter, was very energetic in the womb. She moved all about almost every minute of my pregnancy. Around my third month of pregnancy, I remember feeling a fluttering movement which eventually turned into strong kicks. We thought that she was definitely going to be a boy because the kicks were so intensely strong. Today, Nefertari is a little, petite ball of thunder. She has so much energy!

Seku, my son, has a strong personality too. He was quite active in the womb as well. His personality is also very spunky.

Heartbeat!

Elisa: When I first heard the heartbeat with Nandi, since I had a miscarriage before, I cried and felt very happy. I was really excited and the doctor said, "Well, at this point there's no turning back. We've got a baby coming." It was such an awesome sense of relief. There was no turning back and the baby would be here and safely arrive.

When I heard it with Jair, I felt overwhelmed since it was so real at that point and we had no idea we were becoming pregnant with him. It was such a grounder. All of a sudden we were in this again.

Zaakira: The most fond memory that I have in regard to hearing a heartbeat was when I went to my last weekly doctor's visit during my last pregnancy with my son, Seku. My doctor had arranged for my girls to come in and hear the baby's heartbeat. He gave them a tour of his office and then he allowed them to listen to Seku's heartbeat.

> ❀ **Doppler Monitors:**
> *The baby's heartbeat can usually also be detected as early as 20 weeks with your doctor's doppler monitor, a portable instrument that is held to your stomach and can produce real time sound of the activity in your womb (in this case a heartbeat) through its speaker unit.*

They were so excited they could hardly contain themselves. My oldest daughter exclaimed, "It sounds like a drum at the Afram Parade!" We all laughed and then the girls proceeded to march around the examining room. After my mother marched them out to the waiting room, I found out that I had dilated 4 centimeters. The baby was on his way.

Having the girls there during that last visit was a nice culmination to the pregnancy. It was a wonderful experience for them. They still reminisce about that day.

Lorinda: I was definitely relieved that there was a heartbeat. I was really glad to see that there was a heartbeat to accompany that little figure and I was overjoyed to know that the baby was doing fine.

Michelle: To me, confirmation of a heartbeat signified that everything was okay. During my first pregnancy, I wanted to hear the heartbeat on every visit, be it by ultrasound or Doppler. The sound quickly became my security blanket.

With my next pregnancy, I was extremely timid while awaiting this milestone, given the miscarriage I had recently suffered. During my first ultrasound, it didn't show and I began to cry. Blood work was started to determine if I had a viable pregnancy and all we could do at that point was wait and see. The blood work looked promising, and a repeat ultrasound was performed. Alas, the heart was pumping! We were so relieved. There appeared to have been a miscalculation of my due date and how far along I was. Relief and hope set in.

Ultrasound

This is what your ultrasound experience might resemble, with a technician who will manipulate the imaging device that will allow your baby's activities to be seen on the monitor. Often times the technician will print pictures from your ultrasound for you to keep.

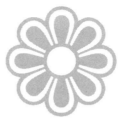

New Parent Glossary

As you proceed through this book and as you proceed through pregnancy, there will be terms that a first time parent (or friend of a pregnant mother) might not be familiar with. The glossary that follows will hopefully assist your navigation through this book and the wonderful experiences of pregnancy and childbirth.

Throughout this book you will see definitions, medical advice and helpful hints in addition to the commentary of the mothers. You can consider this glossary to be an "at-a-glance" reference for some unfamiliar terms you might need to be refreshed on. This glossary continues intermittently for several pages and if it's not here don't forget that the index at the end of the book is where you need to go to find a comprehensive listing of everything covered within these pages.

ABRUPTIO PLACENTA - *This is when the placenta detaches from the uterus before childbirth, either incompletely or completely.*

ALPHA-FETOPROTEIN (AFP) - *This is a substance found in the mother's blood (produced by the unborn child) which is used to detect potential problems with the baby. An expectant mother is usually asked to give blood for the AFP screening between the 16th and 18th week of her pregnancy. It is only a screening test and must be followed up by other tests if blood levels appear abnormal. Your doctor will explain the test when the time comes to give blood and many times even when an abnormality exists in the AFP screening, upon follow-up your unborn child is fine.*

AMENORRHEA - *In your pregnancy, amenorrhea is simply the normal ending of your menstrual cycle or the absence of a period.*

(continued on the next page)

NEW PARENT GLOSSARY
(continued from previous page)

AMNIOCENTESIS - *This is a very common procedure for detecting abnormalities with your unborn child. When circumstances suggest its necessity, this procedure is usually performed between 15 and 17 months. It involves the ultrasound monitored insertion of a needle into the pregnant mother's abdomen and into the amniotic fluid that surrounds your baby. Some fluid is then removed for analysis. Your doctor can give you more information if this procedure becomes necessary.*

AMNIOTOMY - *The artificial rupture of membranes (water breaking) performed by your physician under varying circumstances.*

APGAR SCORES - *The rating of newborn color, cry, respiration, muscle tone and reflex, taken 1 minute and 5 minutes after the baby is born. These scores are a generalized indication of your newborn's well being at birth on a scale from 1-10. Don't be alarmed if your baby is not a perfect 10, it is almost never the case that a baby is at birth. If your pediatrician is not an attending physician at the hospital where you give birth, she will be interested in your baby's apgar scores on her first visit, so record them.*

AREOLA - *The pigmented circular area surrounding the nipple. During breastfeeding it is important for the baby to have the areola, as well as the nipple, in her mouth to make breastfeeding easier for baby and less painful for mommy.*

BELLY WEDGE - *This helpful device makes for a more comfortable sleep for the mother-to-be. It is a support pillow that is "wedged" under the belly to ease the burden of the added weight.*

BRAXTON-HICKS CONTRACTIONS - *These are contractions which "tune-up" the uterus in preparation for real labor. Your uterus is exercising the muscles that will be used when labor finally arrives. These contractions can usually begin as early as 20 weeks into the pregnancy.*

Braxton-Hicks contractions have been described as "false labor" because they have sent many first time expectant mothers hurrying to their physician or to the hospital, only to find out real labor has not yet begun. It is nonetheless important for a woman who is experiencing these contractions to describe them to her physician.

BREECH PRESENTATION - *This is the position of your unborn child when, instead of the head facing down toward your cervix, the child's head is up and its bottom is down. Most babies, if they are not already head down, will move into the proper position as the time for delivery nears. You doctor will discuss options with you if it is determined that your baby remains breech.*

Chapter 5
New Parent Preparation

Parents should begin preparing for their child's arrival into this world as soon as they know the baby is developing in the womb. The forms of preparation can be mental, as well as getting all that will be needed to meet the baby's material needs.

This entire book has been a testament to our mental, spiritual and emotional preparation for the beauty of creation. So, in this chapter we hope to help you with both your preparation as an expectant parent and the preparation for your baby's material needs as well.

Now, if you've just found out you're pregnant, you don't necessarily need to run out and buy everything right away. You do have some time. But, it never hurt to plan ahead.

Michelle: I think my purchases were based on reading because, although I had handled infants a lot, I didn't know what today's baby needed. I also was not very well informed about the rules and regulations as far as cribs were concerned and those kinds of things. So, I just starting combing the baby stores and furniture stores looking and searching for appropriate colors.

And, I was looking for color schemes that would be transitional for either a boy or a girl, since I didn't know what I was having.

I think the best thing for an expectant mother to do is to register because you could end up with a lot of things, such as gifts, that you don't necessarily want or duplicates of things you already have. As far as buying for the baby myself, I really didn't start until I was about 6 months pregnant. There were superstitions involved, in terms of buying things too early and then something going wrong with your unborn baby. If you already had everything for the baby, it would definitely make it harder.

So, at about 6 months I had already decided on furniture color and the theme of the nursery. At that point we ordered furniture. I was blessed, because I didn't have to buy a whole lot. Baby showers tend to bring tons of gifts for babies, so it was just kind of odds and ends that I had to get really.

One of the major things when you're a nursing mom, or you're preparing to be a nursing mom, was trying to decide what kind of bottle or nipple you are going to try and get your baby to use. My first son, Quinn, didn't have any problems going back and forth, but he preferred the nipple that was most like the breast. Once I determined that it made life a lot easier.

Elisa: The first thing I did was call Michelle. I knew she had just had a baby, so she was already adept at all the buying. She told me where to go and where not to go; what stores had good prices and good quality, versus low prices and poor quality. She told me what sorts of things I could afford to go a little bit cheaper on, as opposed to things like furniture, where she recommended that we just go with the best quality. Good furniture will last for a long time through many children.

So, the earliest thing we did, when we found out it takes 12-15 weeks to order nursery furniture, was order the crib and armoire and changing table. I'm glad we did that because it took a lot longer than we had anticipated. We ordered the furniture when I was about 25 weeks. It seemed kind of awkward going in there with my husband, Erriel, because I was showing, but not big and I felt kind of silly walking around. But, that was probably the first thing that got me really excited and I just couldn't wait for the baby to come. I had the anticipation of how the nursery was going to look and which wall to put the crib on versus the armoire. That was when it really hit me that a person was going to come and live in our house forever. And it wasn't going to be just our house anymore, my husband's and mine, it was going to be another person's house and there was always going to be another person around. It was just like a reality check.

And then, after buying the furniture, that's when I decided to start picking out what I wanted for the nursery. Wall colors, prints and stuff like that. So I went to Hechinger's and Home Depot and those types of stores trying to find which colors to use. I finally decided on peach and dusty blue, because I didn't know if it was going to be a boy or a girl. Then I talked to my husband about painting a mural on a short wall. So, we sat down together and drafted what we wanted the room to look like. I told my husband that I wanted feather painting, instead of wallpaper, over a background color. And I thought that I wanted a pale, pale silver, but then I decided on a pale peach and we feather painted with the blue and a darker peach to match everything else in the room. My husband did the mural. The whole thing was step by step, almost every week we did something else, like sketching, then picking out colors, then going to buy the paint and then buying the acrylic paint to paint the mural on the wall. It gave us something to look forward to and something to do in preparation for the baby together. We spent a lot of time, we calculated about 100 hours we spent just preparing the nursery. It was really nice time and, of course, being pregnant I wouldn't play any loud, hard music, so we played lullaby music in the nursery while we painted or talked or sketched. It really was solidifying of the fact that we were going to be good parents and we were going to be caring and that we would transfer all of the time we spent before the baby into the newborn. I think we did a pretty good job of that.

And then, as the weeks wore on and we got the crib and that sort of stuff, I made meticulous lists. I went to Baby Superstore, now Babies-R-Us, about a hundred times and made lists of what to have. I checked these lists with Michelle to be sure of whether I should or should not have some of these things.

I called Michelle one day and asked her, "What are 'oh neesees' and why do I need them." And Michelle said, "What are you talking about?" So I told her it was on the baby registry and I spelled it for her, "o-n-e-s-i-e-s." She started cracking up and said, "those are 'one-sies,' you know the undershirts with snaps on them that come under the babies bottom and snap around the front."

I felt so stupid because I really had no idea. I didn't even know what onesies were, let alone how to raise a child. That was another reality check.

Once we had the baby shower, I checked off everything on my list. And we were snowed in the weekend after the baby shower, so I got a chance to look at everything. I found out what we had and what we still needed. I made another thorough list and as soon as we could get back out after the snow, we shot over to Baby Superstore again. We also decided to get the baby its own credit card so we could keep real close track of how much money we spent just on the baby, as opposed to putting it on our various credit cards that we already had. So we got the baby its own gold card and we put everything on there. I remember that visit. We put things on the credit card that we didn't get at the baby shower, and we got a whole bunch of stuff at the baby shower. Our first visit to the store cost $700. We just looked at each other and said that we couldn't believe how expensive this was going to be.

At the baby shower we got big gifts, like a car seat, diaper genie, layettes, clothes, diapers, some bottles, bath toys, a bath tub, a whole bunch of bath supplies, baby food, etc. I knew about my baby shower, only because it was going to be at my house. And maybe I'm just the kind of person who needs to know things in advance, but I was glad to know so that I wouldn't worry about whether I would go into labor before I had my baby shower. But it worked out really well. I had the shower about 6 weeks before I was due, which was really, I think, perfect timing. It gave me a chance to sort through all the items I got, make my thorough list and go back to Baby Superstore and make returns and exchanges. And all that before I got so big and uncomfortable that I didn't want to go out anymore.

The list I made after my shower contained all the practical

day to day stuff. I needed 7 or 8 more onesies and I needed undershirts that snapped on the sides because of the umbilical cord. I also needed alcohol to swab the baby's navel until the remaining cord fell off and tiny, little-bitty socks and ten things of baby soap. And I even bought baby lotion because I didn't know that you weren't supposed to put lotion on a baby, but luckily our pediatrician told us that on our first visit so we didn't make the mistake of putting it on the baby.

I bought shampoo, a lot of bassinet sheets, a baby wedge so the baby could lay on its side, receiving blankets and diapers. We really stocked up on diapers and they grow through the sizes so fast that I kind of wish we hadn't bought as many as we did, because we ended up having to save some for the next child.

So, by the time we got everything and had the furniture in the nursery, the walls painted, the crib bedding that my mother made, the curtains my mother-in-law made, it had just become such a labor of love and everybody in the family came together and made things. Finally, the only thing missing was a lamp and I couldn't figure out what kind of lamp I wanted, so I remember going all over town trying to find the perfect lamp. We went to 5 or 6 stores and we couldn't find anything. Then one day we were walking past the bagel place and there was a lamp shop there. We went in to check and the first lamp we came across was a little lamp with a teddy bear on it and it was peach, blue, lavender and yellow, which was just right for our baby's color scheme. And it said "Baby" on it, so we bought it.

Zaakira: I did have a list of items to buy, but I didn't actually even start shopping for those things until about 7 months into the pregnancy. Of course you hear the old wives-tales that say you should wait just in case something happens, don't prepare the nursery until 2 or 3 months prior to the delivery, etc.

Most of the things I needed though, I got from my baby shower. I had two showers that year before my first child. They were both surprise showers. I had no idea that they were planned. So, once I went through an inventory of the things I had, I really didn't have to get too much more.

However, I did have a list of things that I wanted, which I had made up somewhere around my sixth month of pregnancy. I was all excited about this nice layette, all the things you're supposed to take to the hospital and all of the things you need at home. Fortunately, even many of the things on that list were given to me as shower gifts.

So, the things that I had to end up purchasing were things that were really for myself. I didn't have to get too much for the baby. I had so many gifts. The thing I enjoyed the most was that I didn't have to buy any kind of lotion or baby care product for my child for the first year of her life. I had so much Johnson's lotion, baby shampoo, Q-tips, Desitin, baby oil, baby bath, bath kits, bath rings. I was also fortunate in that I got a lot of clothes and a lot of people who bought clothes bought them for sizes 3 to 6 months, instead of for newborns so that my child would have some clothes to grow into. They do grow so fast. So I didn't have to get any clothes. I got a lot of onesies, which I was really fascinated with because I had never seen them before.

I got tons of diapers and wipes and things like that. I got a lot of age appropriate toys for newborns and infants. You

New Parent Glossary
(continued from page 62)

CERVIX - *The opening and channel-like entrance of the uterus at the top of the vagina.*

CESAREAN SECTION - *Also known as a c-section, this form of childbirth is by the surgical removal of the child from the womb. A c-section is performed whenever it is deemed safer, by your doctor, than a vaginal delivery. This procedure involves an incision fairly low on the abdomen, near the pubic hair line.*

COLOSTRUM - *Described as "pre-milk, this high-protein, high calorie fluid is produced for a period of time before a woman actually produces breastmilk. Colostrum is the first nourishment the newborn baby who is breastfed will have. Though this fluid is almost transparent and sometimes difficult for the new mother to see, it is there.*
  Colostrum contains the beginnings of the baby's immunologic protection, as well as nutrients and is an important part of breastfeeding. In addition, it aids in the baby's elimination of meconium.

DESITIN® - *One of the more popular ointments to relieve and prevent your baby's diaper rash.*

DILATATION - *The opening of the cervix in preparation for delivery. Your cervix will reach 10cm dilated when your child is ready to be born.*

ECLAMPSIA - *A more severe form of preeclampsia in which siezures and/or a coma could result.*

ECTOPIC PREGNANCY - *This is when the pregnancy implants and begins its development outside of the uterus.*

EFFACEMENT - *Effacement is the thinning of the cervix in preparation for childbirth. It is measured in percentages up to 100%. This process allows for complete dilation and the passage of the child through the birth canal.*

ENGORGEMENT - *This condition tends to occur once a mother's milk comes in. It is marked by full, tender and very hard breasts that can be very painful and difficult for your baby to nurse from. A baby that, at the time of engorgement, is eager and able to nurse is one resolution to this expected problem. An electric, double breast pump can also be extremely helpful to get rid of the abundance of milk causing engorgement. For mothers who don't intend to breastfeed, hot showers or ice packs can help until the engorgement resolves.*

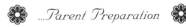
NEW PARENT GLOSSARY

INDUCED LABOR - *Under certain circumstances you and your doctor may make the decision to induce labor, which simply means that your physician will have you admitted to the hospital and your labor will be jumpstarted by rupturing your membranes or administering the medication, Pitocin.*

KEGEL EXERCISE - *This is a series of movements designed to tone and ready the vaginal and perineal areas for delivery.*

LACTATION - *The production of breast milk.*

LET DOWN - *This phenomena is when a mother's milk comes in. It is the actual sensation of milk entering the milk ducts. It can occur not only when milk is produced for the first time, but often also when it is time for baby's feeding or if baby is crying.*

LIGHTENING - *The descent of your baby into the pelvic cavity. Also known as the baby "dropping."*

LOW TRANSVERSE INCISION - *One type of incision made during a c-section, also called a bikini incision.*

MECONIUM - *The first bowel movements of your baby will be Meconium, a sticky substance that is greenish black in color and is the product of the amniotic fluid the baby swallowed while in the womb. A newborn baby should have a meconium bowel movement by 24 hours and several thereafter before normal bowel activity begins.*

MEMBRANES - *These hold the amniotic fluid that the baby rests in until labor and delivery. When the membranes rupture (your water breaks) the baby is usually delivered within 24 hours, to decrease risk of infection to the baby..*

MIDWIFE - *Midwives are individuals trained and experienced in managing the labor and delivery of pregnant mothers. In states where they are allowed to practice independently, these certified practitioners represent a personalized alternative to a physician in low-risk, uncomplicated pregnancies. These individuals practice* MIDWIFERY.

ONESIE - *A one piece undershirt that snaps under your baby's crotch to keep it from gathering and riding up baby's stomach. Onesies can be worn by your baby once the umbilical stub has fallen off.*

know, like rattles and other eye-catching colorful things for the baby to play with. I received a car seat, diaper pails and the whole nine yards, anything that you could want.

The things I had to get for myself were the things that I needed for the hospital visit. Recently, when I've given gifts, I've given gifts for the mom instead of the baby. Things like the little nursing gowns and things that I found I really couldn't live without. Also things like slippers and other little toiletries that you need, especially after the delivery.

Lorinda: Well, before our children were born we kind of made a list of what we needed. We didn't get anything right away, at least for the first baby. But toward the end of my pregnancy, maybe in my seventh month or so, we got a crib. We also wanted to wait until the baby shower and see what kinds of things we would get. Then we just supplemented what we got from the shower with things we needed and didn't get as gifts. For example, we got one car seat at the baby shower, but we wanted one for each car. So, we bought the second one after the baby shower.

Also, people from our church had given us a lot of things, so we had a lot of little clothing items like t-shirts, sleepers, receiving blankets, crib sheets and onesies. But the big items like car seats and the crib we got ourselves. We also had to buy more bottles and those kinds of small things.

The Baby Shower

This could be one of the most fun (and cost saving) times of your pregnancy. Though for your own sake you should recruit a friend or family member to plan it (someone will probably volunteer), there is room for your participation in the planning of your baby shower, even if the time of the shower comes as a surprise to you.

One of the first and most important ways that you and the proud father will participate in the baby shower is to register at a store, such as Babies-R-Us or J.C. Penny. Many stores now days, including the two mentioned, have baby registers. These registers offer a multitude of items that new parents will need in order to be ready when the time comes for the new arrival.

Once you choose a store or two in which you would like to be registered, there will be a registry form that will ask for your name, address, nursery colors, nursery theme (if you have one), due date, etc. You fill out this information so that your completed registry form can be asked for and viewed by friends and family who come to the store to shop for your shower.

You and your mate can then take your registry form throughout the store looking for the items that are listed on the form, most of which you will need at some point after the arrival of your baby. Some of the items included on the register itself can usually include the following (and much more):

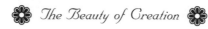
✸ Furniture/Cribs
Armoire
Bassinet
Crib
Changing table
Dresser
Glider

✸ Bedding/Nursery accessories
Blankets
Bumper
Cloth diapers
Crib bedding
Crib sheets
Lamp
Mattress
Mobile
Night lights
Receiving blankets
Sleeping wedge
Waterproof pads

✸ Clothing
Bunting
Gowns
Onesies
Socks
T-shirts (side-snap)

❀ Bath needs
Baby shampoo
Baby soap
Bath toys
Baby tub
Brush
Comb
Hooded towels
Washcloths

❀ Diapers and changing needs
Baby wipes
Diaper pail
Diaper rash cream
Disposable diapers

❀ Strollers/Car seats/Carriers
Baby carrier
Car seat
Car seat accessories
Infant car seat
Stroller
Umbrella Stroller

These are just some of the types of items that might appear on a baby registry. The categories might differ from store to store, but the general items tend to be the same. You will have the opportunity to choose brand names, colors, etc. for

❁

PREPARING YOUR BABY'S NEW HOME

* *Don't wait until the last minute to finish the* **baby's room**. *Paint, decorate and order furniture well ahead of time.*

* **Baby's furniture** *most often will have to be ordered. For the* **crib, chest of drawers**, *and other large items can take as long as 12-15 weeks to arrive. Plan ahead! As far as play pens, high chairs and those types of items go, they will not be necessary immediately in order to be prepared for the baby's arrival at home. However, it is sometimes good to have everything by the time your baby arrives, because newborns require a lot of attention and energy. Keep in mind that you will receive a lot of the smaller items for baby at your baby shower (and some of the larger items depending on your family and friends or whether you will use furniture passed down from other family members). Also,* **Crib** *sheets (6-8),* **blankets** *(6),* **bumpers, crib pads** *(4), a baby* **mattress** *and* **waterproof pads** *(4).* **Bassinets** *can come in handy as well.*

* **Baby t-shirts** *that snap up, rather than pull over, for the ease of taking care of the umbilical remnant that will remain for a while and require your attention. Get a quantity of these shirts (7-10). As with most newborn needs, your baby will go through them quicker than you might imagine.*

* **Baby gowns** *that pull over, with elastic around the bottom. This will be the only type of outfit necessary for a little while, as your baby sleeps a lot (hopefully!) and still needs both umbilical remnant care and constant changing.*

* **Baby socks** *to keep those little feet warm. You will probably need 6-12 pairs depending on how often you intend to wash clothes.*

* **Receiving blankets** *to keep baby swaddled and cozy. 6 will probably do the trick initially.*

* **Diapers** *are going to be a constant need for a long time to come. If you are using disposable diapers, buy a large pack of newborn (60 or so) to begin with. These won't last you nearly as long as you might think! You'll also need* **baby wipes, tissues**, *and* **cloth diapers** *(6) to dry baby's bottom after washing. You will have to do some washing of baby's bottom (in the sink or wash basin) after some of the larger, more runny bowel movements which, by the way, won't phase you at all once you see that beautiful newborn.*

If you are using **cloth diapers**, *you'll need several dozen. Another option is a diaper service.*

You'll also need some means of disposing of soiled diapers! There will be quite a few of them. Either a diaper pail or a Diaper Genie will work fine.

PREPARING YOUR BABY'S NEW HOME

* *A* **baby tub** *or* **wash basin** *will be necessary for baby's baths. Initially when you get home from the hospital, your newborn will not take a bath in a tub until the umbilical remnant falls off. Until that time your baby can be sponged off with baby's new* **sponge** *or wiped with one of baby's new* **washcloths**. *When baby is ready for baths, you'll need* **baby shampoo**, *a* **shampoo brush** *(you should bring home the one used in the hospital after your baby was born.), gentle* **baby soap**, **large bath towels** *(4-6), and a* **bathing head support or pillow** *(many baby bathtubs have a built-in head support). You won't need to use lotion on your new baby right away. Newborn skin is very well moisturized, besides lotion tends to clog their pores.*

* *If you're breastfeeding you'll need a* **breast pump** *for yourself (we suggest the electric double pump),* **nursing pads, nursing bras** *and* **nursing gowns**. *Besides* **bibs** *and the pretty, colorful* **cloth diapers** *to wipe his or her mouth and chin with, baby needs your breasts and perhaps some formula and several bottles (6) for supplemental feeding, father feeding or feeding when you are unavailable.*
 If you are bottle feeding you will need **small 4 oz. bottles** *(10) initially,* **nipples, nipple rings** *and* **caps**. *And, of course, you'll need to find an infant formula that you'll use for your baby. Most of the infant formulas are supplemented with iron, which your baby will need. Sometimes your newborn will make the decision on the kind of formula you use, rejecting one or unable to tolerate another.*

* *A* **diaper bag** *will be necessary unless you plan to never leave the house. In the bag you will carry diapers (obviously), bottles, wipes, tissues, extra outfits and other miscellaneous needs when out with baby.*

* *You'll also need a* **baby carriage** *or* **stroller**.

* *Cotton balls, alcohol, and Q-tips are also handy items that you will use.*

WELCOME HOME BABY!

the items that you select. Couples often spend hours in the stores filling out their registry. The baby registry and baby shower are a wonderfully exciting way to jumpstart your new life with baby.

The person organizing your shower will buy invitations and make sure that everyone is made aware of the stores you are registered in. Another neat thing about the baby registry, especially if you register in only one store, is that it prevents people from getting duplicate gifts. Once a gift is purchased from the store you are registered in, a note is made of the number of such items already purchased and the number you indicated you needed. All in all, it is a neat way to shop without spending any money and, more importantly, it allows friends and family to participate in the miracle you are experiencing.

Fathers Are Expecting Too!

We seldom think of fathers as being expectant. And sometimes for good reason. Number one, they don't carry a growing human being around for 10 months. Mothers have to go through an awful lot. However, fathers too play a rather large role in pregnancy and can have a role to play in childbirth as well.

Fathers have a great deal of responsibility in helping the mother-to-be navigate the dual processes of pregnancy and childbirth. After all, this is the man who provided the other half of the stuff necessary to make a baby (the sperm). Your pregnancy is not a one way street. It is important for the expectant father to know as much about what you are going through in your pregnancy as possible. This is such a tremendous and life changing time that a lack of understanding and a lack of communication can wreak havoc on a relationship; with mother's hormones in flux, focus being shifted from the relationship to the mother's needs with the impending birth of a child, and the uncertain excitement of a new addition to the family.

Now more than ever, there needs to be communication and understanding. The expectant father should be in tune with the terms and unique "lingo" of pregnancy, attend prenatal visits, etc. And, the street definitely does run two ways. Expectant fathers are indeed expectant and have needs that must be respected and understood as well. Participation in bringing a child into the world on either end of the equation is quite a huge responsibility.

So, we recommend that you have this book not only for yourself, but also for the expectant father. In fact, we have decided that rather than simply have a section in this chapter, the expectant father has a chapter of his own.

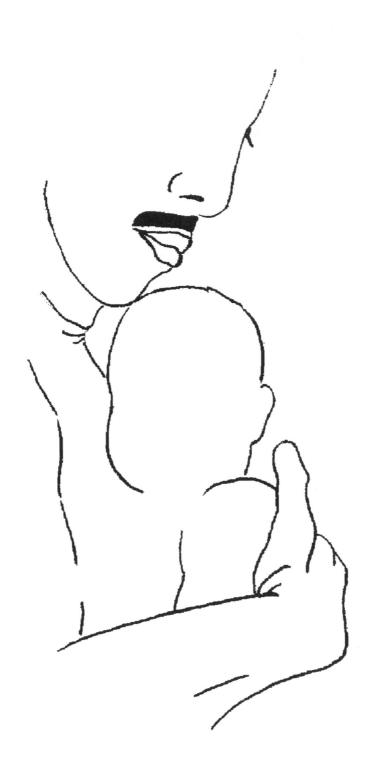

Chapter 6
Fathers Are
Expectant Too!

It is not by accident that this chapter, dedicated to fathers, appears in the middle of a book about pregnancy and childbirth. Fathers truly are a part of the pregnancy process and should be a vital part of childbirth. Fathers are indeed expectant too! So, this chapter is directed toward fathers-to-be, but as with the rest of this book, it should be read by expectant *parents* and those around them who care.

One of the first things to realize is how fathers fit into this whole process. Aside from the biology of making babies and the father's contribution of sperm and genes, his role is actually quite large. Fathers bear the responsibility of bringing a child into the world just as the mother does, only in a different, but still important way.

When the decision has been made to have a child or when this discovery happens quite by surprise, the new parents-to-be should know that this is something that they both will have to get through together. Yes, it is a beautiful time of life, but it is not without its challenges.

First of all, expectant fathers must immediately realize the demands that this new state of being will place upon the mother-to-be. It must be realized immediately, because changes can be-gin to happen almost immediately. A woman's body changes internally in such a dramatic way. Her body begins to work overtime in preparation for this huge life event.

These body changes may very quickly show themselves in the form of fatigue. Naps may become necessary where they previously were not and a few extra hours of sleep may be re-quired. Now this may be something that slightly disrupts the normal flow of MNC (Married No Children) life and is not necessarily of the new mother's choosing. Fathers must under-stand the fact that this is not laziness or always a conscious choice to take it easy (though she deserves it). With the addition of extra blood volume, the sharing of blood oxygen with the new addition in the womb, and the frantic activity of hormones, an expectant mother is bound to be a little more tired than usual. Expectant fathers who realize what is happening, and why, tend to be better equipped to deal with and show more sensitivity to the mother who is experiencing these changes.

> ❀
>
> **ADVICE:**
> *During the course of her pregnancy, the expectant mother's organs will be literally crammed aside to make room for baby, her blood volume will increase by as much as 50%, and she will undergo a multitude of wonderful preparatory changes in anticipation of the child that is developing inside of her. To understand the changes that are taking place is to see the wonder and beauty of them. So try a little tenderness during this time.*

And, as we're sure most people know from the stereo-types that are often presented of pregnancy and expectant mothers, the hormonal activity that the woman must go through is bound to sometimes result, or perhaps often result, in mood changes, very fragile emotions, more frequent tears, etc. In additon, *anyone* who is facing a big change in life might exhibit fear, anxiety, irritation and the like.

Again fathers, the more you know about what the new mommy is experiencing, the more pleasant the experience will be. There may be rough times and times when dad is also dealing with his own emotions, but all in all things will be much more *beautiful* with understanding and communication. And, keep in mind that pregnancy is temporary! You will more than likely miss it when it's gone, though the result of it is even more astounding: your child.

❀

MORE TIPS FOR THE EXPECTANT FATHER:
* *Read as much as possible about pregnancy and childbirth (we probably don't have to tell you that because this book is a wonderful beginning!).*

* *Take into consideration what the mother-to-be is going through and try to be patient, especially if she experiences mood swings. Believe it or not, many times it really is beyond her control and she doesn't mean to hurt you or be mean.*

* *Be tender and loving, showing her that she remains radiant and beautiful even when she doesn't think so.*

* *Occasionally her needs may be a little more urgent than yours. Consider why before getting upset.*

What About Me?

Yes, for the father-to-be, pregnancy is about more than simply how to consider the emotions and changes the expectant mother will have to go through. As we mentioned before, a life change of this magnitude has its effects on expectant fathers as well as mothers.

Expectant fathers very often have worries about the health of the mother-to-be as the pregnancy progresses. Issues of whether or not he will be able to stand the sight of his wife in so much pain in the labor and delivery room; concerns about the growing family's financial outlook; fears about the shifting family dynamic and the responsibilities of fatherhood; anxiety over questions like, "Will I be a good father?" and how the new addition to the family will affect the relationship; and of course, as people shower attention on the mother-to-be, the question of "what about me?" arises.

So as not to leave the needs of expectant fathers by the wayside, mothers-to-be and those who surround the proud parents-to-be should understand that in a sense the mother and father are both pregnant. It is this sense of togetherness that makes the ride smoother.

So fathers should not be seen as ancillary figures in this whole process. And fathers can do a lot themselves to avoid being peripheral spectators.

As fathers-to-be, it is important to be involved in the pregnancy from the beginning. If you are able, attend your wife's prenatal visits and if she doesn't yet have a regular obstetrician, get involved in the selection of a doctor. It should be a doctor and office that you are both comfortable with.

❀

QUESTIONS?

* *Will I be present when my wife is having the baby? (We certainly hope so! This is the 90's and she needs your help and coaching through labor and delivery.)*

* *How can I watch helplessly with my wife in so much pain? (If she can make it through it, you certainly can! Seriously though, the mother's body has spent almost a year preparing for this. Cheer her on coach!)*

* *Will life ever go back to normal again? (No, it will be better than that! Your wife's figure is not permanently pregnant and you now have a beautiful addition to the family. Enjoy the change!)*

For fathers to read pregnancy books like this one, there is more benefit than simply becoming more sensitive to the new mother's needs. In fact, the more fathers know about this process of pregnancy and childbirth, the easier it is for them to be involved in it and the more comfortable they feel. So read and become knowledgeable to help yourself as well as the mother-to-be.

In addition to supporting your mate in her times of need throughout the pregnancy, let her know of your fears and anxieties (Prepare for those times when she may not want to hear a thing about what you are going through, given all that she is experiencing. Tough skin is sometimes necessary.). In those times when your mate seems to be in a good mood and not dealing with her own anxieties and fears, you may find that she is happy to know that she is not alone. Together you may be able to feel better and even when your wife is dealing with her own fears, perhaps it might be good to let her know your fears so that she doesn't feel alone. It might be good for fathers to know, however, that as the due date approaches it becomes less and less appropriate for the father-to-be to expect his needs to assume center stage and gain attention. And, of course, never ever expect any consideration of fatherly anxieties or needs during labor and delivery. What a mistake that would be!

❀

ADVICE:
Labor and delivery are the absolute wrong times to discuss your fears with the mother-to-be! Her needs are the only consideration during this time and for good reason.

Perhaps one of the best ways to get in tune with the beautiful nature of pregnancy and childbirth is to get to know your child. That's right, get to know your child. Though your baby is still in the womb, he or she can hear you read stories and sing songs. As soon as you find out that a child is expected, you can begin to talk to your wife's belly (and your child), sing songs, read books and play music. As your wife gets later into the pregnancy and your baby grows, you may even be able to make physical contact with your baby! With increased movement in the womb, you may be able to tickle a foot or just feel your baby turning and moving around during active periods.

It is also quite natural for a father who is involved enough to sing, read and talk to his child in the womb to also want to be a part of the baby shower. Many baby showers these days are thrown for the proud parents-to-be, not just mothers. Often couples attend these showers as well. It might be a good idea to suggest this to your mate if she has not already thought of it. The occasion can still be a pleasant and special day for her if you're there. In fact, our experience is that baby showers with fathers present and participating tend to be even more special.

There are simply a plethora of ways that fathers can take their

❀

GET INVOLVED FATHER-TO-BE!

* *Attend as many prenatal visits to the doctor as you can. It is especially rewarding and priceless to be there together when you see the baby on the ultrasound for the first time or when you hear the heartbeat for the first time.*

* *Share your feelings and anxieties with your wife.*

* *Read and become knowledgable about pregnancy and childbirth in order to get yourself more comfortable and involved.*

* *Talk, read and sing to your baby in the womb. It is a wonderful way to get connected and even though your child is yet unborn, he or she can hear you and benefits from this stimulation. You can also play soothing and positive music for your baby and baby will hear.*

* *Suggest that the baby shower be for couples and attend it. Gifts for the baby are as important to you as they are to the mother-to-be and don't feel slighted if the mother-to-be gets some pampering gifts of her own.*

* *Participate in the selection of baby furniture as well as the planning of the baby's nursery.*

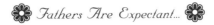

NEW PARENT GLOSSARY

(continued from page 71)

PERINEAL - *A fibrous and muscular area, covered by skin, that lies between the vagina and the rectum.*

PITOCIN - *Generic name Oxytocin, this medication is a hormone that is administered through an IV to induce labor.*

PLACENTA - *The placenta develops on the uterine wall where your fertilized egg has implanted. It produces hormones to assist in the maintenance of the pregnancy, as well as allows the baby to benefit from oxygen and other materials exchanged through the mother's blood supply.*

PLACENTA PREVIA - *This is when the placenta implants over, or partially over, the cervix.*

PREECLAMPSIA - *This is high blood pressure experienced during pregnancy. It can develop between the 20th week and one week after delivery.*

POSTPARTUM - *This term refers to the period of time after the baby has been delivered.*

POSTPARTUM BLUES - *Sometimes a woman will go through a period of depression after the birth of her child. This has been referred to as postpartum blues.*

PRENATAL - *This term refers to medical care and other occurrences that take place before the birth of the baby (i.e. prenatal care, prenatal vitamins, etc.)*

ROOTING- *This describes the instinctive searching for a nipple to suck that newborns tend to do. It is often the signal of a hungry baby or one that simply needs to be comforted.*

SCIATICA - *This is pain along the sciatic nerve which runs along the region of your hip bone. This pain can occur at differing times during pregnancy and usually radiates from the lower back through the buttocks and the back of the thigh.*

SONOGRAM - *Ultrasounds, also known as sonograms, are a safe, painless and very common way to get a good approximation of the date you conceived, whether the growth of your developing baby is normal and a lot of other helpful information.*

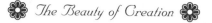

rightful places alongside mothers as proud expectant parents. Fathers don't have to be left out and asking the question, "what about me?"

Your Role in Labor and Delivery

The time to decide what role a father will play in the labor of his wife and delivery of his child is now. A good beginning is attendance at prenatal visits, as mentioned before. The expectant parents should also discuss the logistics of who will be in the labor and delivery room when baby arrives. Many of the more modern facilities that have birthing rooms allow the father plus two family members to be present.

We very strongly urge and recommend that the father be there if no one else is. Make plans to attend childbirth preparation classes with your mate so that you can both prepare for the experience together. Around your wife's 32nd week of pregnancy these childbirth preparation classes begin and last up to 6 weeks, allowing a couple to complete the course roughly two weeks before the expectant mother's due date. Talk to your wife and ask your obstetrician about the classes in advance so that you can make plans to attend together.

Speaking of planning in advance, if you want to be the best support person for your wife that you can possibly be, communicate this to your wife and then the two of you should communicate this to

> **ADVICE:** *Familiarize yourself with the rules and regulations of the labor and delivery ward of the hospital or birthing center where you and your mate plan to have the baby (this can usually be accomplished at your childbirth preparation class). Make plans to be with your mate under all circumstances during labor and delivery.*

your physician. It should be made known that under all circumstances you want to be by your wife's side. If your physician is someone you are comfortable with and you have an honest conversation, he or she should be able to accommodate you. It is not uncommon during an emergency c-section, for the husband to scrub and put on sterile emergency room garments to be by his wife's side during the procedure.

Generally speaking, you can assist your mother-to-be mate through the entire labor and delivery process by bringing her ice chips when her mouth becomes dry (she is not allowed to eat or drink during this time); massaging and applying pressure to her back when she has back labor (something you can learn about later in this book); coaching her breathing during contractions and lending a hand to squeeze or to bite (careful!) during the difficult contractions.

❀
ADVICE:
During a c-section the mother is usually conscious, so your support and reassurance is vital.

Whatever the scenario, a good father and mother-to-be team is very important. Fathers, don't worry about fainting at the sight of blood or breaking into a sweat when the going gets rough. The important thing is that you made the effort to be by your wife's side. And in those instances where your wife is unable to be the first to hold the baby, who better than you?

After the Big Event

After the labor and delivery have gone smoothly and you have a newborn to care for, there are still a few other things to be mindful of. For example, if your wife opts to stay in the hospital for 48 hours after the birth of your new child, will your

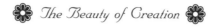

NEW PARENT GLOSSARY
(continued from page 87)

SPOTTING - *This is a way in which light bleeding during pregnancy is described. It can be a little scary, but often nothing at all is wrong, though your physician should always be made aware of any such bleeding. (See the chapter on pregnancy complications for more information.)*

TRANSITION - *This is perhaps one of the most well known stages of labor for its stereotypically raving, pain riddled woman in labor, screaming at the top of her lungs and cursing her husband. It is actually that time during which labor becomes most demanding. Contractions are long and very strong during this time. It is a very intense time and much support is needed. Thankfully it is usually short.*

ULTRASOUND - *See sonogram*

VBAC - *Vaginal Birth After Cesarean. Women who have had c-sections can deliver vaginally in subsequent pregnancies.*

REMEMBER, IF YOU CAN'T FIND IT IN THE GLOSSARY, GO TO THE INDEX IN THE BACK OF THIS BOOK.

pediatrician be able to check on the newborn in the hospital or do you have to contract a pediatrician to fulfill this important task? Will you be staying in the hospital overnight with your wife after the birth? If so, a private room will be necessary providing that the hospital allows spouses to stay the night. Arrangements for a private room must usually be made upon your wife's check-in to the labor and delivery area. And, make sure that you have a change of clothes or at least a tooth brush and a face towel.

And what about your insurance company policy with regard to notification of the birth of your child? Some companies require that notification be made via phone call within 24 hours of the birth, as if you didn't already have enough on your mind. This along with the paperwork to check your wife in, as well as the postpartum paperwork that is usually delivered to your wife's room the day after delivery, can be a little overwhelming if you don't make some plans in advance.

Once the baby is born some fathers choose to make additional decisions. For example, requesting ahead of time to cut the umbilical cord or, if it is a boy, arranging to be present at the circumcision. These decisions should be made prior to labor and delivery. You can speak to your doctor about the necessary arrangements.

Yet another decision that is growing more popular is the choice to exercise a Family Leave of Absence, if you are employed by a company that has this option. Typically this involves the provision for a certain amount of unpaid leave for plan members, including new fathers, to be home with their new family.

Among the other responsibilities that sometimes arise after the birth of your child can be taking care of the portion of the hospital stay that has been billed for the private room (which your insurance may not cover). Sometimes you are asked to handle this kind of cost, as well as the percentage of the hospital stay that you are responsible for personally, before you leave the hospital.

And, of course, in the rush of labor and the impending arrival of the baby, don't forget to have installed a car seat in the car you plan to leave the hospital in. You can't take your baby home without it!

Planning makes everything go smoother. As you and your wife read this book, hopefully fairly early in the pregnancy, make a list of all the phone calls that will have to be made and write down the numbers. Delegate these responsibilities to family members or close friends so that you can attend to your wife and child.

There is more than enough for expectant fathers to do and plan for as the day you've been waiting for approaches. Good luck! We know you'll do well.

Chapter 7
Money &
Your New Family

Even though at this point the full financial impact of your new child is somewhat down the road, money and career decisions are often one of the early considerations for how the coming child will impact your life. Different people handle such an important decision in different ways, but the first priority should be the child. As an expectant parent you'd be surprised at how these types of financial considerations work themselves out when you have a clear focus on what's important in your life.

Whether you decide to go back to work full-time, part-time or not at all, the decision that is best for you and your child is the best decision. Be happy with whatever decision you make and your child will benefit. Whether you hold down your full time job in the home taking care of your child or outside of the home working from nine to five, you are valuable to your family. You might even find that it is a more difficult and rewarding job being a full-time mommy than working outside of the home. Contrary to the ways in which this society tends to view so called "house-wives," if you decide to stay at home, this decision can be equally as important and sometimes more important than going back to work. If no one else values the full range of decisions made by mothers in the best interest of their families, we do!

Lorinda: I wondered if we were prepared financially. I wondered if I could balance my career and family. I wondered how understanding my employer would be whenever I needed to take time away for family matters. As it turned out, after my first child, I went back to work and with the support of my husband and my child-care provider, I was able to balance my career responsibilities along with my family responsibilities.

After my second child was born, I did not go back to work outside of the home, so I was worried about our financial situation. When I decided to stay at home with our children, I also worried about falling behind in my career field. But, I realize how Blessed I am to be able to stay at home and raise our kids. And, as always, the Lord does provide for our needs.

Michelle: It was overwhelming! Having to prepare for a child changed my entire mode of thinking. I wondered if we were financially prepared and I came to the conclusion that you may never be exactly where you want to be. Most times you just do the best you can. My company management was extremely supportive regarding childcare leave. So this gave me adequate time to research and prepare for childcare prior to returning to work. I was also Blessed to find a nanny (live out) through our church.

Financially, I began to worry most about my children's educational needs; choosing and affording what was best for them. My hat's off to full-time mothers! I quickly learned that being at home is the most challenging career anyone can embark upon.

Zaakira: My family has always been a two income family. Prior to us having any children, my husband Hakim and I had a pretty good time and we could do whatever we wanted without worrying too much about money. If we wanted to travel or do other fun things, we could just do it.

When I was pregnant I really didn't want to go back to work and right now I really don't want to be at work. But, I know that the only way we can get all the things we need for our children and accomplish some of our goals, like opening our independent school, is with me working. I have to work.

The ultimate idea would be for me to stay home and I have tried to think of some things that I could do at home. When we were living in our previous home that really wasn't an opportunity where I could do something at home. I wanted to take other children into my home, because I am a teacher and I thought that maybe I could do daycare or something. But, where we lived before I really couldn't do that.

So, I was trying to think of other ways that I could get through this. Luckily, with my first two children I really didn't have to worry too much about paying for sitters, because my children were allowed to go with me to the private school where I was working. They were allowed to go free, which was good because it kind of kept us close to the same financial situation that we had initially. But I still had to work in order to get that benefit.

When my third child came though, that's where we ran into a situation where we are paying mega bucks for daycare. I have to have someone come pick up my children every morning, take them to school, pick them up from half-a-day and bring them back home to me in the afternoon. And that's kind of costly, but it's something that I have to do. But now, luckily I've changed jobs and I don't work for a private school anymore. I work for a public school and they're able to pay me a substantial amount more. That helps.

The financial aspect is always a problem, especially during the summer for me, since I'm a teacher. Those 3 months out of the year are usually a stressful time. We have to do little fun things that are free and that are at home. We save our money and penny pinch a little, but its worth it. You get through the financial worries. It's doable and you just have to do it because it's for your family.

Even with the worry, I do have the best of both worlds. I do work for 9 months out of the year, but for 3 months out of the year I'm at home with my family. That's kind of a good thing.

❀
ADVICE:
As you consider the future of your new family, think of what sacrifices might have to be made in order to meet your goals for the kind of environment you would like your child to grow up in; whether childcare is your choice or will one of the parents stay home?; whether your lifestyle and career are modifiable to less material comfort and more family time if necessary; etc. There are no wrong answers, only what is right for you.

Elisa: I didn't have concerns about my career because I was the kind of person who just assumed I would go back to work. But when I became pregnant, I guess around the second trimester, I realized that I didn't have any desire to go back to work. I was going to do whatever it took, make any sacrifices, in order to stay home and raise my children myself.

I can't really remember a day that the decision to stay home was made, but luckily for me it wasn't even a long, arduous task pondering whether or not to do it. It was just plain that I wanted to be home with our children at all costs. So, my husband and I talked about it and it's not as though we planned or saved ahead. We just decided that whatever sacrifices needed to be made would be made and that in God's Will we would be able to manage it.

Here we are almost 3 years later and I haven't gone back to work. I haven't thought about my career again, though some day I'm sure I will work again. But right now my most important job is with my children.

With money, yeah I do worry about money and I think that I probably worried about money even when we were both working. We didn't have many things to spend it on then though, other than ourselves, and it was easy for me to just be selfish in that way. But, I'm positive that even if I were working now I would still be worried about money, because it's not an issue of me worrying about dollars and cents or caring about big cars and fancy jewelry. I'm more concerned about the well being of my children and their happiness and them having every possibility and every advantage and every opportunity that I could possibly give them.

So even if I were working now, because of the motive for me wanting more money, which is for my children, I have to decide how they are better served. Is it better for them that I keep my career and keep working or spend that time with them doing the job of raising them the best way I know how as their mother? The answer is clear to me, which is why I chose to stay home. I don't care about money so much that I have to drive a Lexus or have diamond rings. I could care less since I'm at home with my children everyday. And, rings and everything else will come and go, but this time with my children is an investment and something that only happens once. I can always go back and purchase tangible things, but with all of the money in the world

I can't regain this time. I cherish every moment with my children and I wouldn't trade it for the world.

That's not to say that I don't respect and understand the decisions that working mothers have had to make. I've been there having to make that tough choice. It's a very personal decision and just like everything else with pregnancy, it's a decision that each individual has to be comfortable with and proud of. I'm just personally thankful for the ability to have the choice. For me there was no real competition when it came down to the choice.

❀

DECISIONS, DECISIONS...

* If both expectant parents have careers or are working, have you begun looking at the childcare options? Good childcare can be expensive, but there are often waiting lists as well.

* If you decide to have childcare, will you have a nanny or a daycare center?

* If you weigh the cost of childcare, is it requiring as much money as one of the household incomes. If so, and you had a desire to stay home, you might as well.

* Will you need to budget to accommodate your new family member and maintain your standard of living? (Babies are expensive, but well worth it!)

Depending on your particular circumstances, there may be a number of decisions you have to make to prepare for your expanding family. Don't panic, you have time and things tend to have a way of working themselves out. The important thing is that you are happy!

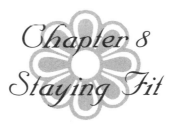

Chapter 8
Staying Fit

Elisa: As a certified group fitness instructor for over 15 years I have had my share of inquiries, questions and comments about prenatal exercise. Luckily in the past decade there has been exhaustive interest and research concerning safe and effective exercises, as well as modifications to existing exercises, for the mother-to-be.

To be nationally certified to conduct prenatal exercise one must participate in courses, workshops and practicals (workouts) every 2 years. I am happy to report that the information has changed for the better over the years! There are so many concerns and points of departure, so I will take them not in order of importance, but in order of frequency.

The first question my aerobic class participants ask me after learning the good news of their coming baby is, "Will I ever get back my pre-pregnancy shape?" The answer is a resounding YES!!! Don't be fooled though. It will take a lot of hard work and even more willpower, but it is not out of the realm of possibility. Actually, some of the people who appear to be most physically fit at my club

---

❀
TIPS:
With some hard work and will-power it is possible to regain your pre-pregnancy shape.

are moms!

While, of course, the composition of your body will not change, the effects of added weight being applied to different areas of your body can change the dimensions. For example, after having larger than normal sized breasts during pregnancy and possibly breastfeeding, the effects of gravity can alter your pre-pregnancy body design.

When I was newly nursing my daughter in a church lounge one Sunday, an elderly woman walked in and was quick to inform me that the baby would "suck" the shape right out of my breasts. I was relieved to learn that she was wrong. However, the added weight of fatty breast tissue and milk would be affected by gravity.

My plan became to attack the real culprit, gravity! I began exercises that would strengthen the muscles that hold up the breast tissue. Since your breasts are not made up of muscles there is no exercise to define them. However, by working the pectoralis major and minor (pecs) you can improve the shape of your breast tissue. They will be held up better, if you will.

Another recurrent question is, "Elisa, will I always have that fatty deposit on my stomach and butt that my mother has?" That question is one that is usually asked in a whisper. Again, the culprit is not your baby or your pregnancy. Remember that you, as a woman, were beautiful and miraculously designed to do just such a task as having a baby. After the baby is born you may have to resculpture your body using techniques that were foreign to your previously taut, firm abdominals, glutes and thighs. Using nautilus equipment or some other weight/resistance bearing machine will surely lead you toward your old self.

Weight training becomes more important as you will not only need to regain shape, but strength in these areas.

A great deal of research by exercise physiologists is proving that spot reduction techniques generally fail without some kind of aerobic activity as an adjunct to weight loss and muscle toning. For example, many of us did aerobics in the 1980's which included leg lifts and intensive glute squeezes at the end of the class. Results were often measured by the "burn" that we achieved but current exercise physiologists have recognized that the burn we aspired to could not give the results we so feverishly hoped to gain. Let's look at those beloved leg lifts that we would patiently do 100 of on a daily basis. On top of the muscles in the leg is a layer of fat. The fat is what makes our leg look fat, not the muscle. So, by trying spot reduction we have succeeded in increasing the size of the muscle, but only to further move out the fat. In order to get rid of the fat, we must burn the calories that feed the fat. That means engaging in some kind of aerobic/cardiovascular exercise.

That leads me to the next question I am frequently asked. "How long can I do my aerobics?" (Or substitute jog, swim, bike, play tennis or some other aerobic activity in this question.) The most important answer is **Consult Your Doctor**. Just as every individual is different, so is every pregnancy. Each of us has special needs that are unique to a given pregnancy. Only your obstetrician is qualified to approve an exercise regimen for you. That may sound textbook and overprotective, but it is your baby's health that is our main concern.

Many doctors will recommend some sort of exercise during pregnancy to help promote the health of both mother and baby. Exercise is important to your physical and psychological health. Barring complications, most women will continue exercising in their preferred manner once they have learned how to adopt modifications that promote safety and effectiveness.

For example, a woman who is a swimmer, aerobics participant, jogger or weight trainer will probably get the green light from her doctor to continue these activities in moderation. An area of extreme concern and caution lies with women who have very sporadically exercised or not at all. If these unconditioned women choose pregnancy as a time to begin a rigorous exercise regimen, their doctor will surely object.

General Considerations for Prenatal Exercise

It is especially important to remain hydrated before, during and after exercise when you are pregnant. Water is still the preferred drink for the soon-to-be mom. Sports drinks are quite high in both sugar and sodium. The last thing a pregnant woman should add to her diet is sodium. Increased salt intake can lead to additional swelling of the feet, hands and even face. The essential electrolytes that are advertised for sports drinks are usually only necessary for professional athletes who train and compete for extreme lengths of time and in extreme conditions.

No mom-to-be should fall into either of these categories. Any discomfort during exercise should be considered an indication to stop immediately. While mild muscular fatigue is normal, pain is not. During weight training exercises the muscle will feel taxed and during any aerobic activity an increase in heart rate is expected. No sharp

---

❀

ADVICE:
There are some home remedies for reducing swelling that might be useful...

* Soak your feet and hands in Epson salt.

* Trace your ABC's in the air with your feet and hands to promote better circulation.

* Keep feet and legs elevated.

* Drink plenty of water and lower your salt intake.

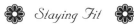

❀
PREGNANCY WORKOUT TIPS

* *Practice stretches at a slower pace and hold stretches a few seconds longer. By doing so, muscles are encouraged to stretch through the full range of motion which promotes elasticity of the muscle (the ability of a muscle to return to its original shape after contraction or stretch). Stretching is likely to be quite soothing for the pregnant woman since some experience sciatica in the lower back, tension in the upper back or pulling sensations near the hip flexor.*

* *Increase the length of warm-up and cool down. Your heart rate and temperature will rise at a more moderate pace. Your body can respond to subtle changes more effectively than rapid fluctuations. If your body has gradually increased in activity, the numerous physiological changes that occur when your heart rate increases will minimally affect your baby. Adequate blood flow, consistent temperature, etc., can be maintained to the baby.*

* *Keep the Beats Per Minute (BPM) slower than before your pregnancy. Remember faster and higher are not always better! Lowering the BPM's will ensure that you will travel at a pace that is more desirable for up and coming moms. Intensity can still remain at a higher level if you feel comfortable and if your doctor has given you the O.K.*

* *The further into your pregnancy you progress, the greater the sensation of breathlessness or the feeling of being easily winded. Of course, this is due to the increased size of your ever growing baby. Decreasing both intensity and impact will most likely become a necessity. Everything you do in some way relates to that little angel of yours. Do both of you a favor and do not exceed your safe and conservative limits.*

❀

MORE PREGNANCY WORKOUT TIPS

* Remember, if at any point (even if it is only in your first few weeks of pregnancy) your doctor tells you it is time to stop exercising, take every precaution and stop! Keep that beautiful little one of yours as the center of your attention and concern. There will be plenty of time for exercising after your bundle of joy arrives.

* Limit lateral movements due to the joint laxity that accompanies pregnancy.

* Do Step-Aerobics only under doctor's advice and at slow BPM with no risers (pods).

* Keep on having fun! Exercise is not only for physical health, but psychological and emotional health as well. For most of us it is a truly fun time of the day. Don't rob yourself of that entertainment by being overly critical of your abilities and expectations.

or dull pain should be experienced. Pregnant aerobic class participants have asked me if the baby is uncomfortable during aerobics. If the mother is uncomfortable, the baby may be also. Keep in mind, however, that your baby is safely nestled in a protective cushion of amniotic fluid. This fluid is probably the most miraculous shock absorber known to mankind. Regular impact does not harm your baby. If, on the other hand, the mother is doing running, high impact full speed on concrete, the impact on the baby will be greater. Surely at this time, the mother will experience some amount of discomfort. The high impact movements may make her belly feel especially heavy and pulled

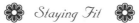

toward the floor. Lower impact modifications will not only improve mom's comfort level, but they will probably allow for greater endurance.

Lateral movement (side to side/right to left) for a woman in her 2nd and 3rd trimesters may be more challenging than it was before. Due to the increased size and weight of the baby, the awkwardness of this new body shape, and the increase in synovial fluid around the joints, moving from side to side is recommended with caution. Balance becomes a very real concern during exercise as the changes we mentioned increase each week. Add to this moving in time with moderate to quick paced music and it is easy to identify the reasons for caution.

Anterior and posterior (front and back) movements are considerably easier to manage since our bodies are more accustomed to walking forward, going up stairs, etc. How often in a day do you grapevine (an aerobics manuveur) right or left to check the mail or climb into bed? Not very often I would assume. We are significantly more adept at traveling up and back. The American Council on Exercise does not contraindicate lateral movements for pregnant women. Caution and common sense would apply however.

High vs. Low Impact Aerobic Activity

There is a great deal of misunderstanding about low or mid-impact aerobic activity. Many people have the impression that high impact is by definition more difficult and more fat burning than low or mid-level options. This is false. It is wholly possible to have a mid-impact workout that is high in intensity and will garner the same cardiovascular benefits. Intensity, not impact, is the key to increased cardiovascular benefits. Fat is still burned at a very significant rate once you have achieved and maintained 40-60% of your maximum heart rate for greater than 20 minutes. The bottom line is that low to mid-impact with mid to high intensity will generate results equal to those of high-impact workouts. So, save your knees, feet and back all of the pressure!

SOME OF THE KEYS TO SAFE PRENATAL EXERCISE ARE:

* Replenish fluids more frequently during exercise than before pregnancy.

*Any discomfort you feel should be considered a sign to decrease intensity or stop activity.

* Allow extra time for warm up and cool down.

Over the past 5 to 8 years the enormous interest in step-aerobics has swept the nation. Since there is little or no impact (it is easy on the joints) and very little lateral movement, it may seem like a preferred method of exercise for the mom-to-be. That may be true for some women, but a few rules would also apply here.

After the first trimester do not add more than one pod (riser). After the second trimester no pods would be the most safe. Balance again becomes the concern of the fitness professional. Keep the Beats Per Minute low to avoid the temptation of traveling around the step too quickly. Try to avoid classes with complicated choreography and weight shifts (center of balance changes from foot to foot, often at half-time). Even if you are a seasoned stepper, the increased size and weight of your belly will change your ability to move around the step freely.

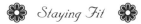

Modifications for the Expectant Mother

Following you will find some visual guidance to suggested modifications for stretching and muscle conditioning. It is recommended that you discontinue abdominal work and leg stretches laying flat on your back at around 16 weeks. Don't worry there are plenty of safe, effective and fun alternatives.

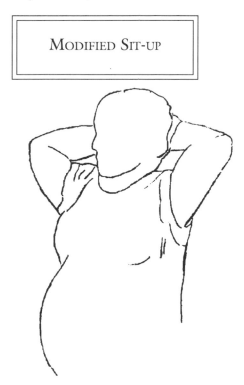

MODIFIED SIT-UP

Modified Sit-up starting position: The expectant mother can stand with her back to a wall and her hands behind her head. From this position the pelvis should be tilted or rolled upward and the upper torso (shoulder area) should move toward the belly in a way similar to the motion of a sit-up performed while laying on one's back.

MODIFIED SIT-UP (OBLIQUES)

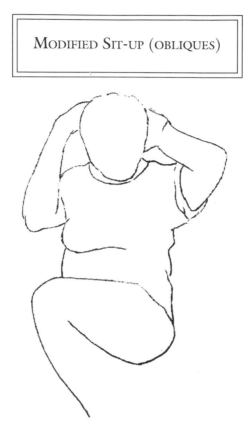

Modified Sit-up end position: The expectant mother should again balance herself with her back against a wall. With the pelvis rolled upwards, one knee should be lifted while the opposite shoulder and elbow are moved downward as if to meet the elbow to the knee.

MODIFIED PUSH-UPS

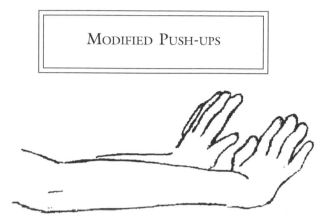

Modified Push-up for the triceps: With hands placed against a wall and fingers facing the ceiling, the expectant mother should do a push-up motion against the wall, while standing upright.

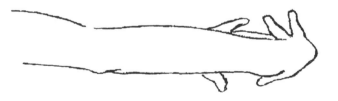

Modified Push-up for pecs (chest): With hands placed against a wall and thumbs inverted toward one another, a push-up motion should be performed against the wall, while standing upright.

INNER THIGH

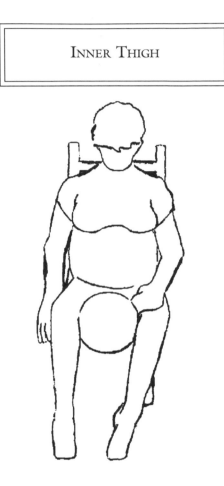

Inner Thigh: While seated comfortably, the expectant mother should place a rubber ball between her knees and gently squeeze inward, as if trying to bring the knees together.

GLUTEUS (BUTTOCKS)

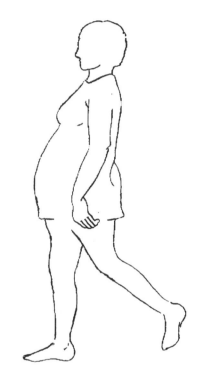

Gluteus (buttocks) ending position: Standing, while supporting herself with a chair or wall, the expectant mother should lift one leg backward and upward. The knee should remain relatively straight. Legs should be alternated.

OUTER THIGH

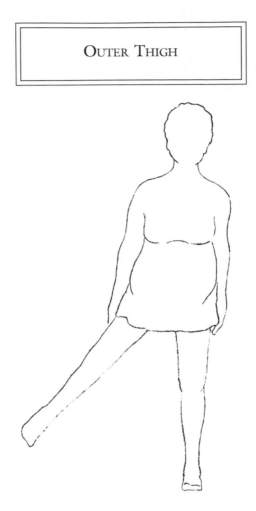

Outer Thigh ending position: Standing, while supporting herself with a chair or wall, the expectant mother should lift one leg directly out to the side of the body and up. The knees should remain relatively straight. Legs should be alternated.

LOWER BACK STRETCH

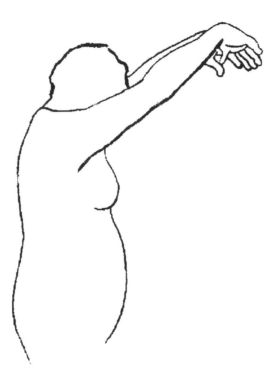

Lower Back Stretch: The expectant mother should roll her pelvis upwards and roll her shoulders down toward her pelvis, creating a "C" shape.

POSITIONS THAT MAY RELIEVE
SCIATICA AND GENERAL BACK
PAIN

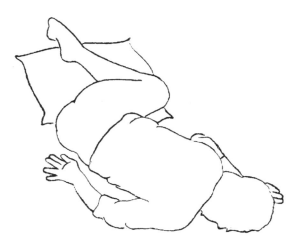

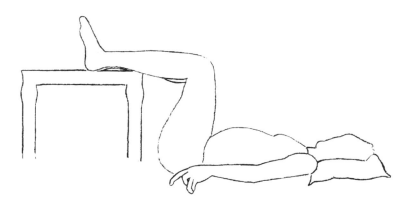

✽

CHILDBIRTH PREPARATION CLASS

Before your big day (or night) arrives, you have an excellent opportunity to refresh yourself on the type of information that you will pick up in this book and to learn even more information. Chances are you will also get the chance to practice breathing with your partner, visit the hospital labor and delivery rooms, brush up on what to expect in labor and during childbirth, etc.

This wonderful opportunity is your childbirth preparation class. These classes usually last 6 weeks, beginning around your 32nd week of pregnancy. They are an opportunity for the expectant parents to have questions answered and shake off some of the jitters of anticipation, while gaining new ones as the reality of labor and delivery are brought into a clearer focus.

Not only will you gain a wealth of new information—with regard to breathing techniques, relaxation techniques, a real tour of the place where you will be doing the real thing—but you also get a refresher course on the immense and sometimes overwhelming amount of information that you've had to grapple with since you found out you were pregnant.

* Childbirth preparation classes are usually 1 night a week for 6 weeks.

* Expectant mother and father (or other coach) are encouraged to attend together.

* You receive good information, reminder sheets that guide you through labor and delivery, and some free samples of baby products just to name a few of the benefits.

* You get a hospital tour, from the check-in process to the actual labor and delivery rooms.

* You meet nice people who have one great big thing in common with you: they're expecting too!

* And you get an opportunity to share with other expectant parents what a great resource and source of inspiration this book has been so that they may buy it and recommend it to friends and family!!!!

Chapter 9
The Wait Is Over,
Here Comes Baby!

All the preparation, all of the anticipation of nine or ten months comes down to one day. Labor and childbirth are both the culmination of pregnancy and the beginning of an entirely new life; new life not only for the baby, but for you too!

Don't Forget The Bag!

Zaakira: I had slippers, two robes and two nightgowns since I only stayed overnight after the baby. I also had the undergarments that you typically put in your bag. Me personally, I had to wear socks. I put about 4 pairs of brand new white socks in my bag, because I get cold easily and I don't like anybody to touch my feet. The doctors wanted to take them off and I was like, "I don't think so."

So, the socks, which were mandatory for me, and I had safety pins and hair supplies, even though I purposely had my hair braided because I didn't want to look crazy after I gave birth. I had 2 oufits to wear home depending on my mood. I had a real casual outfit and one that was slightly more dressy, because I knew we would be taking pictures and things like that. I was going to visit my mother-in-law on the way home.

And I had little things that I would need for my personal care. There's a lot of bleeding after childbirth, which a lot of people aren't aware of. I think I had everything I needed and I was real satisfied with what I had. I took books

> ❀
>
> **Tips:** *You'll need a hospital bag packed in advance with clothing for you and baby, as well as various other items you'll need while in the hospital. This bag is both convenient and necessary. Pack it before labor begins.*

and I even took my thank-you cards that I hadn't had a chance to write for people who had given us gifts. I had paper for the list of things that I wanted my husband to finish that he hadn't already finished prior to the delivery of the baby. I had my address book so I could call people while I was there waiting for people to visit. I made calls to announce the birth of my child to friends and family.

I also took little dry snacks like banana chips and little pretzels, because after you eat and the cafeteria closes you're hungry. So I had things that I could munch on in my room and that was basically it.

Lorinda: I had gowns for me, nursing gowns. So, I guess I had 2 gowns and a robe, slippers and panties. And for the baby I had a couple of outfits, little sleepers and a little winter suite for him to come home in. I also had diapers and t-shirts. Of course I also had a comb and other cosmetic stuff, a little make-up here and there, curling irons, that kind of stuff.

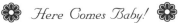

❀
WHAT'S IN YOUR BAG?

What follows is a list of items that you might consider placing in your hospital bag. Prepare your bag around the 36th week of pregnancy and customize it to the needs you anticipate having. Have it waiting and ready for a possible excited rush to the hospital or your obstetricians office. Good locations for your packed bag (to avoid the forgetfulness of over excitement) are the foyer closet, by the front door, and in your car. Feel free to use this list as your personal checklist.

☐ *Your copy of* <u>The Beauty of Creation</u> *(this book!).*
☐ *Your "Goody Bag"*
    - A stopwatch or wrist watch with a second hand for the purpose of timing contractions.
    - Pen and paper to record the time of contractions.
    - Socks to wear in case you get cold feet (literally).
    - A focal point of some sort to focus yourself during contractions (a favorite photograph, stuffed animal, etc.)
    - Lip balm for dry lips during contraction breathing.
    - Tennis balls to relieve back pain during labor.
    - Any other useful items for the time of labor and delivery.
☐ *Camera and film*
☐ *List of phone calls to be made (family, friends, insurance company, etc.) and who is responsible for making them. You and your husband should have delegated these responsibilities amongst reliable friends and family.*
☐ *Magazines*
☐ *Toiletries*
☐ *A couple of gowns (nursing gowns if you will breastfeed).*
☐ *Slippers*
☐ *Bras (nursing bras if you will breastfeed).*
☐ *Lotion*
☐ *Toothbrush*
☐ *An outfit for the new mom to wear home.*
☐ *An outfit for the new baby to wear home, including baby cap, socks and t-shirt.*
☐ *A receiving blanket.*
☐ *Sanitary pads, though the hospital will provide you with extremely large pads and funny looking fishnet panties, which are actually necessary for the post-partum bleeding.*
☐ *Snacks to supplement the 24 hr. gourmet (just kidding) hospital meals.*

*And, finally, make sure that you and your husband have remembered to install the car seat ahead of time. First time parents, especially those in the throws of last minute panic, may need some time to figure out the proper installation of the car seat. (The car seat should be in the middle of the back seat, **facing backwards**. This is the safest way for the seat to be positioned.)*
Good Luck!!!!!!!!!!

Elisa: Our prenatal childbirth class instructor gave us a list of things to take into the labor and delivery room so that we could be prepared for any of the challenges of labor. These things were kept in a bag inside of the hospital bag, which was called the "Goody Bag." For example, for lower back pain we had tennis balls to massage my back; lollipops to suck on in case of a really dry mouth or for the sugar if you get really tired; and a couple of pairs of socks in case your socks get wet or soiled or anything. But your feet are still cold from pushing and working

---

❋

ADVICE: *It is a good idea to have a bag within your hospital bag, which I call a "Goody Bag." This bag should contain various items that you would like to take into the labor and delivery room. Such items would include things like socks, stopwatch, pen and paper to time contractions, lip balm, lotion or baby oil, etc.*

---

so hard, so brand new socks. I remember thinking, "I am never going to use all of this stuff. This is alot of stuff." But I used every single thing in that Goody Bag either during labor or after the baby was born. Some of the other things in the Goody Bag were magazines and I remember thinking during labor that I wasn't going to use these magazines because, 'I am in labor!' I didn't read them during labor. But, the next day after I had the baby, when they made me use the bathroom I was so stressed out because I knew it would hurt to go to the bathroom. So I took all of those magazines into the bathroom with me trying to get my mind off of it. I ended up using them that day after the baby came.

The Goody Bag also contains lotion or baby oil so that your husband can rub your back or anywhere that's sore and lip balm because of all the panting and blowing you do during lamaze type breathing when your lips get really dry. I also had my stopwatch, a pencil and a piece of paper to chart what time my first contraction was and monitor throughout labor. During my first pregnancy, since I didn't know I was in labor, I was so excited when my husband got home and we could get the clock out and write out everything, to see if it was the real deal. I still have that piece of paper.

In the regular bag I was really meticulous and I wanted it to be so perfect. I went out and got new nursing nightgowns for myself. Nursing nightgowns are very important so you can easily nurse the baby in the hospital. I got a robe and new house shoes and everything.

My first baby was born in February, so for Christmas my loving husband gave me an adorable little piece of luggage that was paisley, a light pale gray, and tiny enough just for my things and the newborn's things to come home in. And it was such a thoughtful gift. I remember thinking, 'he is so wonderful to buy a gift like this.' I packed everything away in that bag. My toiletries, my outfit to go home, my nightgown and nursing pads in case you get engorged in the hospital. For the baby I packed something to come home in and little undershirts that snap and socks and a little coat and a receiving blanket and a big blanket because it was winter.

With my second child, because I had a 15 month old at home I was really concerned about what would happen with her when I was away. So, early in the pregnancy I tried to prepare things for her so that I wouldn't have to do it at the last minute. Like every time I went to the store to buy something for the unborn child, I would buy her a gift or two and stockpile them away. I'd buy little Sesame Street videos or books or stickers or balls, farm animals and the like.

I guess in total I ended up buying her 15 little things and I am so happy that I did because I also brought 1 or 2 gifts with me to the hospital in my bag. That way the first time she came to the hospital we could give her a gift from the baby. She was just so happy to get a gift from the baby and give a gift to the baby as well.

When we got home from the hospital I knew she would also be a little taken aback because the baby would now be in her house. So the first thing we did as soon as we got home—all of us, my husband, my daughter and our new son—was go into our bedroom and let my daughter open her first gifts at home and we watched a Sesame Street video that was an hour long, while I nursed the baby. And we all just ate lunch, up there together, that my mother had prepared. I think that was a really important bonding time. There is a picture of all of us sitting there and whenever I see it I almost cry. And whenever I see that video I think about it because I'm glad I was able to think ahead enough to make that transition comfortable for my daughter. We were still doing things all together, including her things that she liked to do. And the baby, her new brother, just kind of slid right into the groove of our family and it was really a calm, pleasant transition.

From that point, everyday I tried to ween her off. I'd give her a little something and she wasn't really expecting anything. It's not like every morning she woke up asking for a gift. But, just sometimes if I felt like she wasn't getting enough attention or I needed her to be distracted so I could do something for the new baby, I would give her a coloring book or something and she would be so elated.

So all of that stuff was in and related to the hospital bag. Wow!

Michelle: My husband says I overpack, but I took my baby book, a couple of gowns, a pair of slippers, nursing bra, nursing pads, lotion and other toiletries, a baby "take-home" outfit, a receiving blanket, a little baby cap, a camera and a couple of books.

Reality Sets In: Memorable Moments of Childbirth

Elisa: My most memorable with my second child, Jair, was that since I had been pushing for three hours and I was so exhausted and they finally got me into the operating room, I was thinking that they were going to cut me. I was still pushing with all of my strength trying to get him out because I did not want to have another c-section. All of my attention was focused on pushing. I kept thinking that if I push hard enough and if I push long enough they won't cut me, they'll respect that I've got to get him out.

I was crying because with my first baby, Nandi, I had a c-section and the recovery time left me somewhat sore and immobile for a while. So, thinking about this as I was struggling to deliver my second child vaginally, with a 16 month-old daughter waiting at home, I was so upset at the prospect of my daughter not being able climb on me and jump on me and just play the way she had become accustomed to for 16 months. I was just torn up over the effect that this would have on her and I knew I would miss her too. Staying in the hospital for 3 or 4 days was not an option.

So, while I was being taken to the operating room I was pushing and crying and telling my husband not to let them cut me. I even told my obstetrician to please not cut me. Luckily she was a great doctor and hung in there with me.

Finally, I saw people start crying and screaming and I heard the anesthesiologist say "The doctor said stop pushing, the head is out." I had a relief, an unexplainable relief, and I was thinking, "I did it, I actually did it! All this work and he's here safely." It was a wonderful feeling.

With my first baby, Nandi, what was really so memorable was how quickly she arrived, because it was an emergency c-section. You kind of work toward 10 centimeters dilated or work toward being able to push and your mind is in a state of 'Okay, I'll get to 7 centimeters dilated, then I'll get to 8, I'll get to 9, I'll get to 10 and then I'll be a mother.' But, with Nandi we went from 7 centimeters to a baby. I know we were already there and I should have been more mentally prepared to be a parent, but it just happened so quickly that I felt responsibility and fear and excitement and joy and all of those things more quickly than I could have imagined.

Lorinda: With my first child, Shawyn, it was a planned cesarean, so I didn't know what to expect. However, being that it was planned, everything was kind of mapped out and calculated. I guess the worst part was getting the epidural and being in that little tight ball they want you to be in. That was hard.

So, basically we arrived there that morning and we just waited. Then we went into a room and soon after they gave me the epidural and we went into the operating room. I remember my husband, Alan, saying that the hardest part for him during that time was watching them give me the epidural.

The whole time it was incredible because I knew that my baby was going to be born and we were going to take this baby home. But, in that whole time it felt really different since it was planned. During the actual operation, of course, I couldn't see anything and I couldn't feel anything either.

I relied on my husband to tell me what was happening. So he just described it to me. He said that they actually had to get on my stomach and push the baby down. So that was the first birth.

The second one, I actually went into labor. My water broke at home and I didn't really realize it. I knew something was different, but I felt like I had just passed my mucus plug. But, when we went into the hospital they said that my water had broken and I was having contractions, though I didn't really feel them.

So, I was in labor and it was progressing. I was that way for maybe an hour or 2 hours but my labor stopped progressing. That's when they gave me Pitocin to induce labor. After that it took about an hour and very, very, very intense contractions were kicking in. My doctor actually left the hospital. I guess she didn't think things would progress as fast as they did. So, they were paging her and I was pushing and they were telling me not to push. But I was pushing because I couldn't help it at all. You know it's hard to stop that urge to push.

I was in a lot of pain, because I didn't get an epidural. I guess everything progressed too fast. But now that I think back it might have been because my doctor wasn't there to order one. In any case, I didn't get an epidural so it was very, very painful and very, very intense. And I just remember them trying to hold it off. I mean, I know they were waiting for her, but it was like I just couldn't stop it, so I said someone is going to be here to deliver this baby.

I really don't know how long it took the doctor to get there after they started paging her, I just know that it seemed like it took forever. I just remember my labor nurse looking very...not worried, but she knew that the baby would be here any minute. I could see in her face that she was like, "Where is the doctor?" I couldn't understand why we had to wait for the doctor to come. I knew that there were people there who could deliver it.

The nurse even showed me the head and she knew that the baby possibly could come on the next push, so she was looking and whispering to the other people, "Where's the doctor, where's the doctor?"

The reality was that the baby had arrived in this world and that he depended on us for his every need. I loved our baby from the moment I knew I was pregnant, and when he was actually born, the love I felt was so much stronger. At the same time I felt fearful because I didn't want anything to happen to him. I wish that I could protect my children at all times. Having faith in God helps to take away those fears.

Michelle: My most memorable moment was hearing my son, Quinn, cry for the first time. Quinn was an emergency c-section and that day I had a 2:30pm appointment with my obstetrician. They kept me there probably for an hour and a half running tests and doing the neo-natal monitoring. My doctor wanted me to go to the hospital, but she was very calm and cool about it. So, I went home and ate some left-over dinner and when I got to the hospital they did another ultrasound before they decided to go ahead and deliver. Once they made the decision, I delivered probably within an hour and a half, because my obstetrician was concerned about his breathing. So, from my appointment at 2:30pm, Quinn was born at 6:19pm that same day. It was rather quick.

Because of the c-section, when they finally pulled him out, he didn't cry initially and my husband wasn't answering my questions about how our baby was doing because I guess he was in shock. So there were a couple of seconds of silence. Those minutes of waiting for a cry seemed like hours. Then he cried and it was the most beautiful thing I had ever heard. When they handed me my newborn son, I began to cry. He was so precious. I held him for about 15 minutes (I think???) and they whisked him away. And away went my husband with the camcorder. I don't think I saw him for another hour.

With Blake, my second child, I was scheduled for delivery at 7:30am on November 5th, 1997 and I was reading Quinn a bedtime story the night before when my water broke. So Blake decided he didn't want to wait for his appointment he wanted to be born early. Of course, I couldn't go into labor because of my fibroids, so we left the house at about 9:00pm that night and Blake arrived into the world at about 11:47pm.

Zaakira: Watching the baby grow, I became worried the bigger the baby got. I worried about the pain of labor and delivery and the unknowing aspect of it. You don't know exactly what it's going to be like. In the hospital a woman next to us was screaming and screaming and I said, "Oh Hakim, what happens when I get to that part?" But I never did.

When we got to the point where my husband cut the umbilical cord, there was a finality to the pregnancy and I was a little sad in that there was a separation after carrying my daughter for 10 months. It was time to begin a new life together. Life changed. I can't explain how wonderful it feels to finally meet someone who you have grown to know intimately.

IT'S TIME!

full dilatation

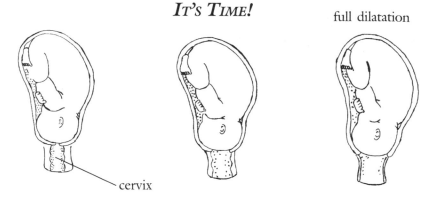

cervix

YOUR LABOR WILL PROGRESS IN PHASES, AS YOUR CERVIX DILATES IN PREPARATION FOR THE DELIVERY OF YOUR CHILD.

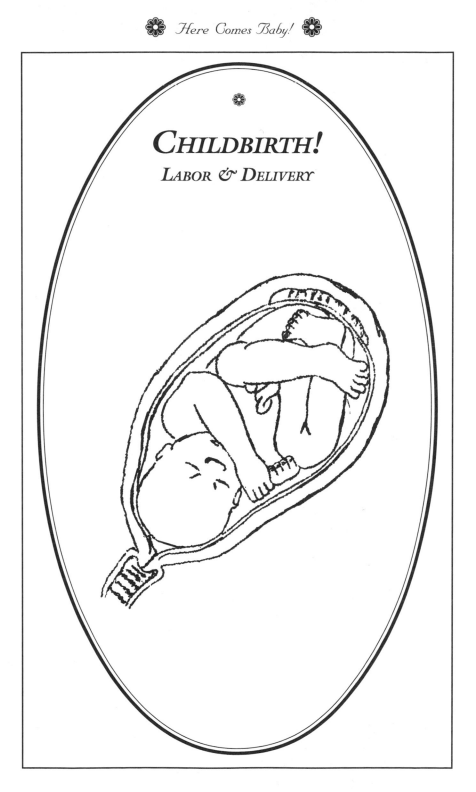

CHILDBIRTH!
LABOR & DELIVERY

❀

BEFORE THE "REAL" THING

Labor has been built up to be much more dramatic than it is in real life. Make no mistake that your labor, and even more so your delivery, will be one of the most fantastic events of your life. However, it is a rare occasion that the labor scenario plays out as it does on television, where the expectant mother is enjoying a normal day and then out of nowhere comes a contraction that forces her to grab her belly and scream out, just before she is hurried to the hospital by her excited husband just in time to deliver the baby. Of course, all of this has had to happen within 30 minutes from beginning to end to fit within the time slot of the sitcom of which this family is a part. Neither is it often the case that the expectant mother is instantly hit with her first contraction and is thrown right away into a frenzied series of shouts and demands directed toward her husband or anyone else in her vicinity.

In real life, nature is much more orderly and patient. Before "real" labor starts you have a warm-up called **prelabor**. Prelabor in some respects is a part of early labor and is characterized by:

* LIGHTENING - This is when the baby moves its position so that its head (in a "normal" presentation) descends into the pelvic area. This is also referred to as the baby "dropping," an early sign that labor is not far away.

* ENGAGEMENT - This is when lightening has occured and the baby's head is fixed in position in the pelvis. Engagement usually occurs about 1-4 weeks before labor begins in mothers who are expectng for the first time and your physician can tell you whether your baby has engaged by doing an internal exam. At this point in your pregnancy you will be seeing your doctor about once a week (after week number 36).

* EFFACEMENT BEGINS- This is the thinning of the cervix, measured in percentages (0-100%). Effacement occurs in preparation for the passage of your baby through the cervix (it allows full dilatation).

(continued on page 136)

❀

LIGHTENING & ENGAGEMENT

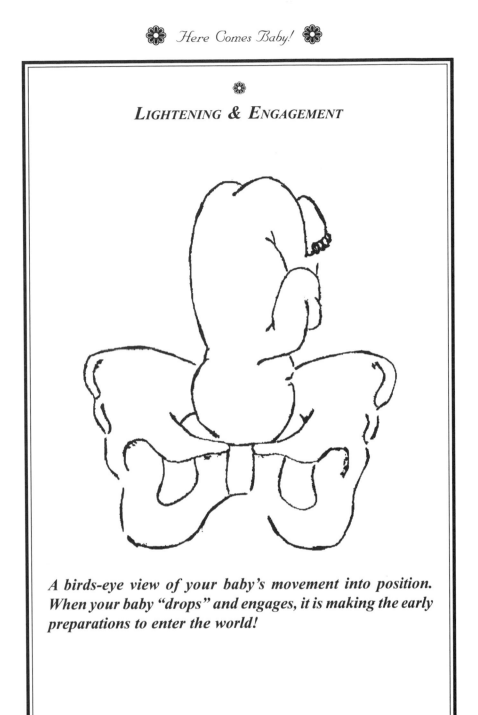

A birds-eye view of your baby's movement into position. When your baby "drops" and engages, it is making the early preparations to enter the world!

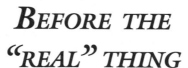

BEFORE THE "REAL" THING

Other signs of prelabor are:

* If you suddenly have the need to wash the car, clean the entire house or build a new wing onto the baby's room, this could be a sign that you are in prelabor.

* You may also experience increased pressure in the pelvic area and the rectum.

* A "bloody show" is a sign that you are in the warm-up phase for the real thing. A bloody show is a mucousy discharge which indicates that the mucous which previously plugged the cervical opening, has given way and may appear in the vagina as white, clear or slightly blood-tinged.

As if the warm-up of prelabor isn't exciting enough, some expectant mothers experience **false labor**. False labor is characterized by:

* Irregular contractions that usually last less than 30 seconds. They follow no pattern in terms of time between them and their duration.

* These contractions also have a tendency to abate if you walk around or change your position.

* The pain of these contractions is just in the lower part of your belly.

Don't be embarrassed if false labor sends you and your husband dashing off to the hospital after a frenzied phone call to your obstetrician. Sometimes during the exitement of the whole experience, it can be difficult to distinguish between false labor, Braxton-Hicks contractions and the real thing.

However, the more you know the easier it will be. Stay calm and everything will happen in time.

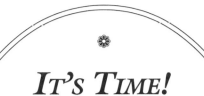

IT'S TIME!

Don't worry, the baby isn't just going to pop
out right away. You will progress in stages, the three stages
being labor, pushing and delivery, and delivery of the
placenta. Perhaps the most popular aspects of this process (aside
form seeing your baby for the first time and feeling the relief of
delivery) are the **three phases of labor**: Early, **Active** and
Transition.

A question that we imagine is also on your mind is "**when do
I call the doctor?**", *so we'll address that first.*
* "WHEN DO I CALL THE DOCTOR?" - *The first answer to that ques-*
*tion is whenever you are in doubt or concerned. If you have concerns
about your signs and symptoms and you need some guidance, whether they
are positive symptoms or complications, call your doctor! Don't worry about
being wrong or embarrassed, just call.*

1) *If your* **water breaks** *or you detect a leakage of amniotic fluid,
call your doctor. Your baby is now out of its protective liquid cushion and the
general practice is to go to the hospital and await the beginning of labor or
induce labor if it has not occurred within 24 hours. With the rupturing of
your membranes (water breaking), the chances of infection increase for
your baby. 24 hours seems to be the standard of a reasonably safe window
for your baby.*

*Usually, when your water breaks, contractions are not far
behind.*

2) *When your* **contractions** *have begun and have established
a regular pattern of increasing duration and space between
contractions, you should begin timing them. When timing
contractions and the question arises of how far apart your
contractions are, you* **time them from the beginning of
one to the beginning of the next (minutes).** *As a
general rule, when your contractions are on average* **5
minutes apart** *and last* **around 60 seconds**, *it's
time! Your doctor will give you his or her specific
instructions.*

3) **Bleeding** *other than bloody show,
call!*

IT'S TIME!
EARLY LABOR

Your day has come and your labor has begun!
Early labor tends to be the longest and least rigorous phases of labor, so relax and try to rest. It is not time to go running to the hospital yet or call your doctor, unless there is reason outside of the normal activities of early labor. Early labor can last for several hours.

Light **contractions** *will begin and tend to be* **30 to 45 seconds long** *and* **5 -20 minutes apart***. They may not be precise in this pattern, but generally close enough to be recognizeable as a pattern. In the beginning they may be so mild they are barely noticeable except for their consistent timing. It differs from woman to woman.*

Eventually the contractions move closer together, become longer in duration and more intense toward the end of this phase. Your doctor will give you a milestone at which to call, usually around 5 minutes apart and 45 - 60 seconds in length.

During this time, your cervix is dilating and effacing. When you go to see your doctor, he or she will appraise you of your progress. Early labor will usually take the mother-to-be up to 3 centimeters dilated.

You may be full of anxiety and anticipation when early labor begins, but you should try to stay calm and go about your usual daily routine, staying close to home. Find something to keep you occupied. You might go for a walk or watch television. If you're hungry you should eat a light snack, but don't eat too much. Chilbirth is a process that will demand all your energy, including the energy your body would use to digest a large meal. You might consider cooking a few dinners to store away in the freezer. Not only will this pass time, but it will come in handy once baby is home and your time is limited.

If your labor begins at night, try to get some sleep. The contractions won't let you continue sleeping when it's time to go.

❀

It's Time!
Active Labor

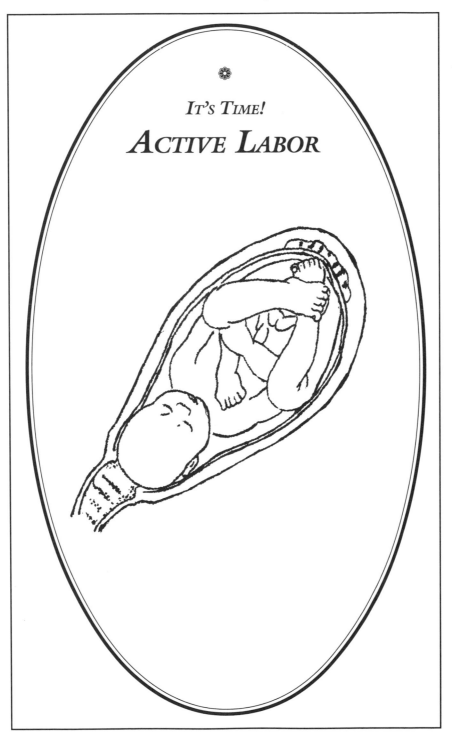

IT'S TIME!
ACTIVE LABOR

You're getting closer to actually being able to really say, "it's time!" You will probably be at the hospital now. Once you enter the active phase of labor, your contractions become more frequent and stronger. Sometimes women may get a little discouraged during this phase of labor. It is getting harder, you've been at it a while by now and you've got less time to rest between contractions.

However, hang in there! You're almost there. This phase of labor usually lasts anywhere from 2 to 5 hours. By this time, your obstetrician will probably have told you to come to either her office or the hospital. Your **contractions** *will usually be* **2 to 4 minutes apart,** *lasting* **45 to 60 seconds,** *though there still may be some variation or slight irregularity in the timing. You and your baby are really starting to work now!*

Your cervix will go all the way to 7 centimeters dilated during the course of this phase. Though you may be feeling very uncomfortable, be encouraged! Those tennis balls in your Goody Bag might be helpful now for the backache. Your husband (or other coach) can help you ease the discomfort.

You can start your breathing exercises now and may need ice chips for your thirst and dry mouth, as well as those socks that you packed just for the occasion.

When mom is wearing an external fetal monitor, there is also a monitor which coach can watch to see the beginning, peak and ending of contractions. This allows teamwork between mom and the coach, so that coach can tell mom when contractions are beginning and direct the breathing. Most importantly coach can reassure mom when she is at the peak of a contraction and on the downside as well. It helps to know that it's almost over.

At this point, if you need medication, you can remind your physician. He will evaluate your progress and get the anesthesiologist if everything is a go.

WHEN YOU NEED MEDICATION

The beauty of childbirth is not measured by how much pain a woman can endure. Therefore whether or not you need or use medication is simply a matter of choice, not an indication of what kind of mother or woman you are. Let your physician know before your labor and delivery that you might want anesthesia during this time. There are several types of medications to be discussed before labor between expectant parents and the doctor. At this time, epidural is an ever more popular choice.

REGIONAL ANESTHESIA

*An **epidural block** is a very common form of anesthesia during labor in which, upon the doctor's orders, a anesthesiologist will inject a local anesthetic into the epidural space (the space that surrounds the spinal cord) in the lower back area. Very often, the mother-to-be is asked to sit upright on the bed, tuck her chin to her chest and curl up into as much of a fetal position as she can manage, curving her back and giving the anesthesiologist good access to the area where he or she will make the injection. A catheter can be left in the injection site to allow periodic infusion of anesthetic as needed during labor. Fetal monitoring will also be required when an epidural block is administered, since it may slow fetal heart rate.*

Epidural blocks are very safe and, though they do not take away all of the pain and rigor associated with labor and delivery, they are helpful for some women who need assistance getting through this time. They may, however, limit your ability to push when the time comes, which sometimes results in a c-section. This potential drawback happens less often and is limited by the ability of the anesthesiologist to monitor and control your epidural through the catheter left at the injection site. When the time comes to push, the epidural infusion is stopped.

***Spinal anesthesia** is another option, but a lot less popular than it was years ago. The anesthetic in this case is injected directly into the spinal canal. It can't be given until the very last minute before delivery, because it prevents pushing. There is also the risk of headache, sometimes severe, with spinal anesthesia. Nausea and vomiting may also be a concern.*

With regional anesthesia, drops in blood pressure can occur, therefore you will be monitored for blood pressure and also are likely to have a blood oxygen monitor on you finger.

*There are a few other forms of anesthesia you can ask your physician about, which are also options for you. Be sure to have this discussion **before** you go into labor. When you are in labor and at the point where you feel you need medication, it is likely too late for you to get it.*

❀

IT'S TIME!

TRANSITION

This is one of the most infamous and demanding phases of labor. It is stereotypically known for the ranting lunatic who is giving birth while cursing everyone around her. This is a stereotype, however. Not every woman handles transition in the same way and though some women are exhausted and lose control to some degree, others experience only the intensity of the increased work load.

*During transition **contractions** intensify, lasting from **60 to 90 seconds**, often with less than a minute between them. Your cervix will dilate the final 3 centimeters and arrive at the 10 centimeter dilatation point when baby is coming.*

There may be a tremendous urge to push, but hold on until you're given the okay. Understandably you might feel like you can't take anymore at this point, your legs may tremble or shake uncontrollably and fatigue may hit you like a brick wall, but relief is right around the corner.

During the transition phase, the husband or other coach becomes most important. They should try to keep the mother-to-be calm and have thick skin themselves. Coaches have to be strong during transition, realizing that it really is all about the mom-to-be. Your feelings as a coach must not come into play here if you have been insulted by an exhausted mother-to-be at her wit's end. Grin and bear it! Comfort the mother-to-be anyway and do what she asks of you (as long as it is within reason.)

Any breathing techniques that have been learned and/or used are needed now more than ever. At the end of this phase you can begin pushing once you are given the go ahead. Hang in there!

❁

IT'S TIME!

DELIVERY

*Push! Push! Push! You are in control now.
The light can be seen at the end of the tunnel and the light is
your baby. Your hardwork has payed off! You are in the home-
stretch. Delivery is the second stage of childbirth. You are through
labor now. You may even feel rejuvenated. This stage is variable from
mother to mother in terms of the amount of time it takes. It may be as
short as several minutes or as long as a few hours. Your* **contractions**
*will be more regular and manageable than they were in transition,
usually around* **2¹/₂ to 5 minutes apart** *and around* **60 seconds or
slightly longer.**

*The contractions are your helper now more than at any other
point in the childbirth process. Your doctor and nurse will be giving you
instructions at this juncture which will be important for you to follow.
Everyone will also take ques from you as to when you are able to push longer
and when you need a rest.*

*Your baby will crown first and the doctor and your coach will be
able to see the top if its head (in normal presentations). You may request a
mirror or one may be offered to you as well, but you'll likely be too busy
concentrating on pushing and resting in between.*

*Occasionally, if you have urine in your bladder or excrement in
your rectum, these may be pushed out during your pushing. By no
means should this be a source of embarrassment nor should you impede
your progress by trying to prevent such things from happening. This
is a very natural and beautiful process and these things are seldom
given a second thought. In fact, they are sometimes expected.*

*And once the head is out, the rest happens in a flash. Here
comes baby!*

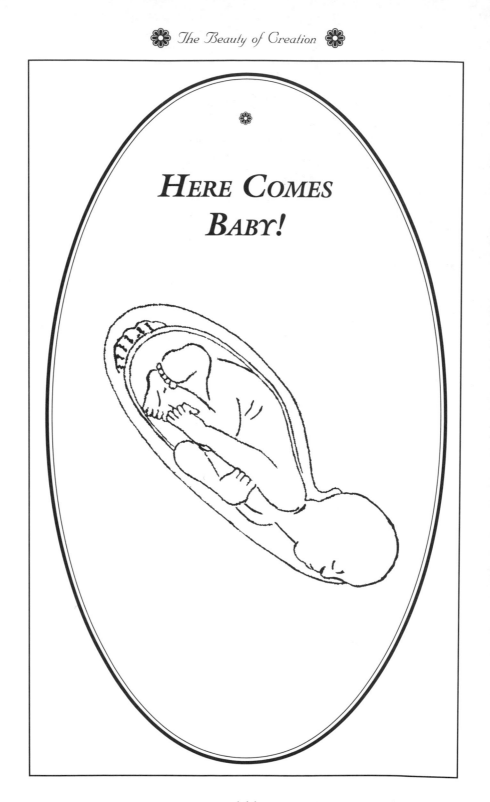

HERE COMES BABY!

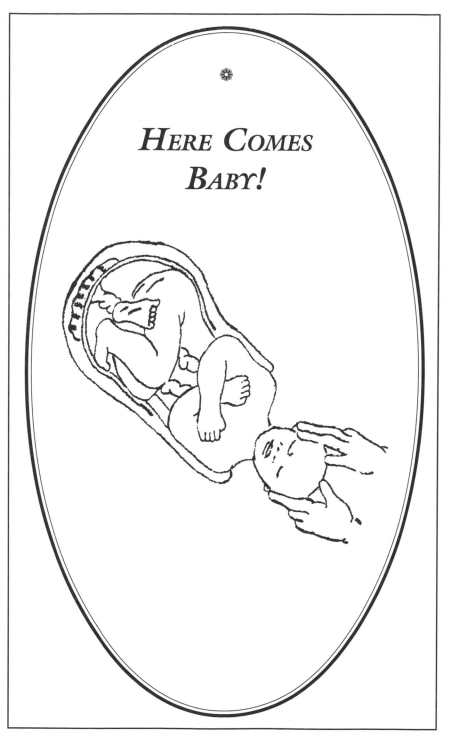

HERE COMES BABY!

Your Baby At First Glance

Don't be alarmed if when your baby is first born he or she is not your vision of the soft skinned, smiling, cooing child you imagined. Childbirth is a process in which a life is moving from a liquid internal environment, through the rigors of childbirth and into the outside world. Sometimes this has a temporary effect on your baby's appearance. Blood from delivery; a cheesy substance covering baby, called the vernix caseosa coating; swollen genitals and puffy eyes; a fine hair covering various parts of the baby's body other than the head, called lanugo; and a head that seems a little distorted, are all potential characteristics of your newborn that are temporary and natural. For parents of color, your child might be of a lighter hue than you expected, another temporary thing which changes over a couple of days as your baby's color begins to come in.

Then again, your baby may come out just as you expected. Chances are that either way that baby is going to be the most beautiful thing you have ever seen! Don't feel guilty, however, if you're a little taken aback by any temporary "funniness" about your newborn's appearance.

What Is This Stuff?

That cheesy looking substance, called the vernix caseosa, that some newborns have covering them is a protective coating that your baby wore in the womb as an insulation from months resting in amniotic fluid. The swollen genitals are often seen in newborns as a result of the mother's hormones. There may even be a vaginal discharge or milky secretions from the swollen breasts of both males and females. It is all normal and temporary. Don't worry!

YOUR LAST STAGE
OF CHILDBIRTH

Your long odyssey of pregnancy and childbirth is just about over. In fact, you may not have even thought much about this 3rd stage of childbirth. Don't worry, a few small contractions and pushes and it will be over.

What is this 3rd stage? It is the delivery of the placenta, frequently called the "afterbirth." Aside from your help, your physician may massage your uterus by pressing down on your abdomen to assist the expulsion of the placenta.

Once the placenta has been birthed, your physician and nurses will clean you up and perform any stitching that may need to be done.

You've made it and your new life begins now. Get some rest and be very proud!

CONGRATULATIONS!

Joy! Joy! Joy!

Elisa: When my first child was born, I was proud of giving birth. I had joined an elite club. Now when I see another mother I feel true camaraderie and sisterhood, like we both know what it's like in the trenches. Sometimes, right after I gave birth, I would swear another woman—sometimes older, sometimes not—would nod at me with a knowing glance as if to say, "Congrats! You did it girl!"

For the first time I stopped downing myself over stupid little things. My baby was perfect and therefore, by association, so was I. I learned quickly how to really love myself, no holds barred.

Michelle: With Quinn I was very alert and given that I was a high-risk pregnancy I felt a great sense of relief. I just felt as though a miracle had happened. Quinn made it against the odds and it was really indescribable.

With Blake, I was a little out of it and I remember that it seemed like it took forever to get him out. But unlike the moment of silence when Quinn was born, Blake came out screaming. It was just pure joy. Indescribable happiness.

Lorinda: When my children were born I was very, very happy. I was praising God. They were healthy and I just thought they were the most beautiful little babies I had ever seen. So, I was very thankful.

Zaakira: You know it's so funny because when my first child was born, I remember feeling really happy and exhausted. But, I also remember this really insatiable hunger. I wanted to eat. I was very hungry. So, my concern for the child was to tell my husband to follow her and make sure she was okay, but I neeed to eat, I was very hungry.

I was also really shaking. I have had it with every child I have had. It's this really uncontrollable shaking and I don't know what that comes from. But, when all of my children were born I felt Blessed and very happy.

Zaakira's Natural Childbirth

Well, I just generally thought it would be the best way to go. So many things you hear tell you that every time you take any kind of substance into your body while you're delivering, there is a possible chance that the child will get some of the substance or drug into their system. The baby is still a physical part of you at that point. I was always concerned about that.

At that last moment after carrying the child for so long, I didn't want to take a chance where something could go wrong because of the drugs. Besides, I really wanted to just try it on my own, which I basically did. I never had an epidural or anything like that. I was really basically able to breathe through my contractions. It was very painful, I won't say that it wasn't. But, I was able to focus and try to get through the contractions, breathing it out.

I also used something called counterpressure. My contractions came in my back area so I constantly had my fists balled up, or a ball, and I would counterpress the area where the contractions were. It kind of helped me, even if it didn't physically, mentally I thought I was doing something. And it helped having my husband there.

I always got to 7 centimeters and I would beg for drugs. I would be saying, "Please, somebody give me something." But it would be too late then. The baby would be crowning. And that was the crucial point because it would become very painful at that 7 to 10 centimeter time. It was the transition point and that's when I would beg for anything. I told my doctor if I ask you for something just ignore me, I'm going through transition.

However, 2 times out of my 3 pregnancies I did get something. I got something called Demerol. They gave me one-fourth of the dosage required. I really didn't want it, but at that point I had been pushing so much that my cervix was swollen. They really wanted me to relax. They coaxed me into taking the medication, because I thought I was superwoman. But, just to relieve me they gave me the Demerol. I was too tense toward the end when I really needed to be concentrating on pushing.

Alternative Childbirth Methods

Natural childbirth involves the utilization of breathing techniques and relaxation to reduce the pain of labor and delivery, rather than medication. There are several different methods, 2 of the most popular and well known being Lamaze and the Leboyer method.

Lamaze is a breathing based method focused on understanding the changes that occur in contractions throughout labor and delivery and adjusting disciplined breathing techniques accordingly. Leboyer, on the other hand, is more focused on how the child's entry into the world takes place. It believes in bringing the child into a more friendly environment where lights are dimmed to near darkness, there is silence, the umbilical cord remains attached for a period of time to allow the child a smooth transition to breathing, a lukewarm basin of water awaits, etc. As you can see, especially with Lamaze, these alternative methods have contributed to the way that most childbirth situations are handled in general.

Homebirth is another alternative birthing method chosen by some expectant parents. As the name implies it involves having your child at home or another more home-like alternative location. Midwives play a significant role in this option. It is based on bringing both the expectant parents and the child through labor and delivery in a more comfortable, friendly environment where they are the focus of attention and have some measure of control. It is focused on birth as a life event that should be shared in a home-like environment and not treated like a disease or disorder within a hospital, with potentially harmful tests and monitoring.

There are numerous other alternative childbirth options that, if you are interested, might be right for you.

Midwives and Midwifery

Midwives have changed over the centuries. Not only are they very knowledgeable and caring people who have the experience of having delivered a lot of babies, but today many midwives have had extensive training as Certified Nurse Mid-wives. Of course, this is to say anything negative about those individuals who have directly entered the midwifery profession. Certified Nurse Midwives can offer primary health care to women, as well as gynecologic and maternity care. They are specialists in pregnancy and childbirth. In many states Certified Nurse Midwives have the authority to write prescriptions for many medications necessary in the process of pregnancy and childbirth.

It is recommended that an obstetrician be involved if your pregnancy is high-risk or complicated. In many hospitals, Certified Nurse Midwives are able to practice as well, giving you the opportunity to utilize your personal relationship with your midwife, while at the same time having the back-up of the hospital and physicians.

Just Be Happy!

Pregnancy and childbirth are unforgettable times in life that should be happy and filled with good memories. Make safe, sound decisions that are good for you as expectant parents and enjoy!

❀

INDUCED LABOR

There are circumstances under which a judgement is made between the expectant parents and the physician to induce or jump start labor, as opposed to waiting for it to start on its own. This decision can be made for many reasons concerning the health of either the mother or the child. (These will be addressed in the chapter on "Complications of Pregnancy & Childbirth")

One of the common means by which pregnancy is induced is by the use of the medication, Pitocin (oxytocin). Pitocin is a synthetic version of a naturally occuring hormone in your body, oxytocin. The Food & Drug Administration no longer allows the use of Pitocin on an elective basis, so voluntary inductions without medical reason are rare.

When a woman is already in labor and labor is not progressing for whatever reason (again, some of these reasons are discussed in the "Complications of Pregnancy & Childbirth" chapter), labor can be enhanced by several techniques.
* If her membranes haven't yet ruptured, they can be artificially ruptured, a process called amniotomy. The doctor uses a rather simple looking, slender, hooked tool called an amnihook to reach through the cervix and snag the membranes, which causes the amniotic sac to open (your water to break). Sometimes Pitocin may still be necessary once this is done.
* Pitocin will be utilized. The nurse will set up an intravenous (I.V.) infusion and gradually increase the amount of medication to get the desired results. With Pitocin, your labor may be shorter and a bit more intense than if it occured on its own.

In cases where a woman's membranes have ruptured, but contractions have not begun, walking may be a way to bring on labor. If contractions haven't begun within an alloted time frame, Pitocin may be used here as well.

There are also occasions when a woman will schedule an induction. The decision to induce is made between the expectant parents and the doctor, and then a time is scheduled for the woman to come into the hospital (usually very early morning) and she will be administered Pitocin to begin labor.

Do not worry! If you have to induce, the only excitement that will be missing from the process is that of labor beginning while you are at home. You will still experience the stages of labor, except for the mild onset of early labor that usually occurs with labor's natural beginning. To prepare your cervix for labor, sometimes a hormone based gel, prostaglandin gel, is administered to your cervix to "ripen" it, or prepare it for dilatation. You are still having your baby.

Chapter 10
"Real" Birth Experience? Having a C-Section

Almost all women, except those with special circumstances going into a pregnancy, prepare to have a vaginal delivery. Most expectant mothers are so prepared for, or fearful of, the stereotypical panting, puffing and pain of vaginal delivery that they give no thought to the possibility of a cesarean section (c-section).

Part of the reason for this lack of forethought is that c-sections are often wrongly categorized as not being "real" birth experiences. Also involved is the fact that there are definitive indications that let you know in advance that a c-section will be necessary.

Elisa: I was so confident, and overly confident I think, that I was going to have a natural childbirth because I was fit and I was young and I was strong. Honestly, I didn't even read the chapters in the books about c-sections. During childbirth preparation classes I only half heartedly listened during the c-section part because I didn't think that was going to be me. So, I was unprepared for a c-section because I was so overzealous about having a vaginal birth, which was actually silly of me.

It seemed like the pushing with the delivery of my

second child, Jair, made it feel like there was something natural about me being his mother and getting him out and being ready to accept him by the natural force of nature. With Nandi, my first child, I had an emergency c-section and it was as if I had no control. I felt very inactive in bringing her here, so that when she did get here so quickly I felt almost inept. It was kind of like I wasn't properly prepared or competent to handle her.

Another thing that was memorable about the c-section was that I was in so much pain from the c-section because mine in particular was bad. It was not because c-sections are bad, mine was just flawed. I was also very disoriented because of the medications and things. I remember actually feeling guilty because when I first saw her I couldn't hold her since I was too busy being stitched up.

INDICATIONS FOR CESAREAN (EXPLAINED FURTHER IN CHAPTER ON COMPLICATIONS):

* *Cephalopelvic disproportion (baby's head and mommy's pelvis are not a good fit)*

* *Fetal distress during labor*

* *Abnormal fetal presentation*

* *Active maternal herpes*

* *Failure to progress in labor*

* *Placenta previa (the placenta is blocking the cervix)*

* *Abruptio placenta (the placenta is separating from the wall of the uterus before the baby is born)*

* *A fetal or maternal condition or illness that makes a vaginal delivery too risky*

* *Mother is 2 or more weeks overdue and uterine integrity is weakening*

* *Prolapsed umbilical cord (the cord is preceeding baby through the birth canal)*

* *Maternal hypertension, diabetes, or kidney disease, any one of which may be uncontrollable or make vaginal delivery difficult.*

In retrospect, a c-section doesn't make childbirth any less amazing or momentous or any less a Blessing or gift, its just different. I don't think that people should feel like they gave in, chickened out or took the easy road by having a c-section. If anything, I think mothers that have had c-sections have gone above and beyond the call of duty by getting cut open for their child. Its like the ultimate sacrifice. I really think that only a mother would do that.

❀

TIP: *Today, even in situations where emergency c-sections are necessary, fathers are allowed to be with mom in the operating room and she is conscious.*

Michelle: I really didn't have any preconceptions about c-sections. My first day was really hard due to an allergic reaction to the pain medicine. But I was up and around pretty quickly. I feel a lot of that had to do with all that needed to be done with caring for my newborn son.

Now, about one year later when I opted to have my fibroids removed, I was told it would be like another c-section. That was a lie. It was very painful and recovery was very slow.

Lorinda: My first baby was born by planned c-section and I didn't expect it to be over so quickly. I also didn't expect the level of pain afterwards. I delivered my second child vaginally, but I was surely prepared for a c-section.

Michelle: In my opinion, c-sections aren't any less rewarding than vaginal births. I don't feel slighted one bit by the fact that all of my future deliveries have to be by cesarean section. After all, the ultimate goal is the safe delivery of your child.

❀

A Glance At A Cesarean Section

If you have a planned cesarean you will make your scheduled trip to the hospital, get checked in and prepped for your procedure. If you are already in labor, you will be prepped and moved to an operating room. In many hospitals the expectant father can scrub, put on surgical gowns provided and meet you in the operating room, if the procedure is being done with the mother-to-be still conscious. We recommend this where it is allowed. Coaches are needed during a c-section as well, to comfort and reassure.

Through the I.V. that has been setup, you will receive a general anesthetic or pain medication. If you were previously in labor and are conscious during the procedure, the anesthesiologist will have given additional epidural medication. A urinary catheter is also installed.

Mom-to-be is prepped and scrubbed and can actually choose to have a mirror setup when baby is emerging or simply get progress reports from her husband. As the procedure begins, it is important to reassure mom. She should feel no pain, only pressure. If she feels pain, the anesthesiologist and obstetrician should be made aware.

There are two options for the kind of incision the obstetrician will make, one is vertical and the other is horizontal. Both incisions are made low on the abdomen into the uterus, near the pubic area. In fact, the horizontal incision is sometimes called a "bikini cut," because it is generally just below where a bikini line would be. This horizontal incision tends to be less painful and heals better, aside from its aesthetic benefits. The bikini cut or horizontal incision is currently the most popular incision, except under special circumstances.

There may be pulling in conjunction with sucking sounds, as the procedure is performed. Incisions will be made through your skin and outer tissues, as well as through the uterus. There will be additional pulling and pressure as the baby is delivered. There should be no pain or feeling of sharp poking or cutting. And then, after a relatively short period of time...

Welcome baby! Once the baby is delivered, mom can see the baby briefly before they place baby under the heat lamp for warmth, clean baby and do weights and measurements of baby. At this point stitches and/or staples are used to close the incisions. Usually the interior incisions are closed using stitches that will dissolve on their own, while the outer incision will be closed using either stitches that will dissolve or staples. This process will probably take around 30-45 minutes and again, you should feel no pain.

After a complication free stay in the recovery room, it's off to your room. One thing that should be known is that your recovery might involve some measure of pain and discomfort. Though you will be encouraged to be up and walking within 12-24 hours, a c-section is not a "blow-off" procedure. It is major surgery. You will need to arrange for someone to be at home assisting you for a week or two once you leave the hospital, in order to make your recovery easier. If you intended to breastfeed, you can still do it with some adjustments, such as pillows to support the baby and protect your incision. You will receive thorough instructions from your doctor.

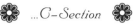
✻
VBAC (VAGINAL BIRTH AFTER CESAREAN)

After a woman has had a cesarean, all hope is not lost for future vaginal deliveries. Your future pregnancies can still result in childbirth by way of vaginal delivery. In fact, women who have had c-sections with the horizontal (bikini incision), officially termed a low transverse incision, are encouraged to attempt labor and very often succeed in vaginal delivery.

* For those mothers who have only had a c-section and think it less threatening pain wise than actual labor and delivery (or those who have had both and felt the c-section was much easier), you don't have a choice of an elective c-section. Your physician will not perform a c-section if it is not necessary.

* An additional worry that some women have is whether or not their uterus will hold up during labor because of the scar from their previous cesarean. With women who have had a low transverse incision (95% of c-sections now) and no permanent health conditions that made the c-section necessary the first time, a complication free vaginal delivery is possible.

If you have to have a c-section, be assured that your experience of childbirth is just as real and valid as anyone else's. There is no reason to experience guilt. You should rejoice in the fact that you were able to bring a child into this world, who grew and developed in your womb.

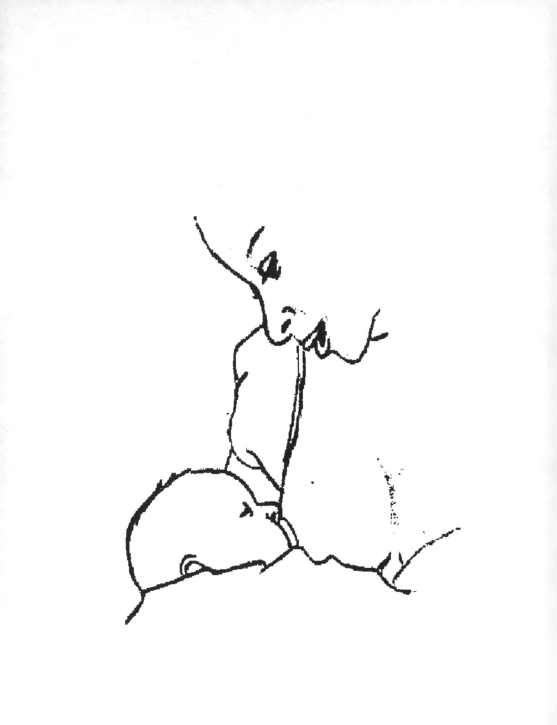

Chapter 11
Mommy's Milk...
Does a Baby Good!

One of the most important obligations of new parents is to make sure that their newborn family member receives the best possible nourishment to thrive and develop into a healthy child. Growing numbers of mothers in the United States are joining the world's mothers in providing the best possible nourishment a newborn can have, mother's milk.

Breastfeeding is another of the miracles that women experiencing the beauty of pregnancy and childbirth will have a chance to participate in. However, few women are told that it may take a considerable amount of work for mother and child to become proficient at breastfeeding. While it is natural, it still takes practice and is not always as simple as raising your baby's head to your nipple. Even so, it remains a very rewarding experience. The body produces a system which, all by itself, is capable of completely meeting the child's nourishment needs for months, and depending on the preferences of the mother and the pressures of society, years.

Not only is the decision to breastfeed a nutritionally sound one, but it has a host of other benefits. Mother's milk helps to build a child's immune system for protection against illness and the act of breastfeeding itself is often soothing to a child who is in pain or sick. For the mother, beastfeeding helps the uterus to shrink back to normal size after childbirth. And, for the mother and child, a special bond is formed during breast-feeding. It is another part of the beauty of creation.

Michelle: I was determined to nurse due to the beneficial effects to my child, but friends shared negative experiences. Fortunately, this only made me more determined to be success-ful. The benefits of nursing are numerous. My children are rarely ill, which I attribute in large part to nursing.

When I began nursing I was hoping everything would go properly (the baby would latch, milk production would be adequate and the pain minimal). Initially it was an adjustment, but in the end it was hard to give up. I can remember one incident, which was our first outing—we attended a festival. While out, I didn't nurse my son at the normal intervals. By the time we arrived back home, he tried to nurse and couldn't latch on. I looked at my boobs and they were swollen, red and hard as a rock. I panicked and we

❀

ADVICE: *Engorgement is a condition that tends to occur usually when a mother's milk first comes in. It is marked by full, tender and very hard breasts that can be very painful and difficult for your baby to nurse from. A baby that, at the time of engorgement, is eager and able to nurse is one reso-lution to this expected problem. An electric, double breast pump can also be extremely helpful to get rid of the abundance of milk causing engorgement. These pumps can usually be rented from a hospital or a lactation consultant.*

It can even happen with new mothers who don't intend to breastfeed. Hot showers or ice packs can help until the engorgement resolves. One home remedy is soak absorbent baby diapers in hot water and lay them across each breast to ease the discomfort. To avoid en-gorgement when baby is not with you to feed, take your pump along.

phoned a lactation consultant, who advised us to come over immediately and pick up a hospital rental pump. Her further advice was to go home, run hot water on two pampers, and use them as hot compresses for my breasts, drink a glass of wine to relax and hook up the pump.

When the milk began to flow it was unreal. The relief was almost immediate. Of course, I had to discard that milk, due to the wine content. But once all was said and done, my son was a happy camper.

Needless to say, I kept the pump. My husband would come home from work and see me hooked up to the machine, looking like a cow, and just laugh. I decided to store the milk I was pumping for future use once I stopped nursing. You would open our freezer and plastic bags of frozen milk would come tumbling out.

When you're breastfeeding you're giving your baby something no one else can. It also gives you private time with your baby to examine little fingers, toes, eyes, etc.

Elisa: Breastfeeing is something that I would recommend for every mother who is physically able. Not only is it a tremendous headstart toward a healthy life for your child, but it is also a time where you can get to know your child. You get to look at those tiny fingers gripped in a fist around one of your fingers. Those eyes stare intently into yours as the baby suckles or they slowly close as your child drifts off into a comfortable sleep in mommy's arms.

It really is a bonding time. And it's not only when your baby is hungry that you will breastfeed. When your baby is hurt or uncomfortable, your breast can be just the right thing to calm him or her down.

Zaakira: With nursing I was sitting there trying to figure out how to get my child to latch on. When she finally did, I was doing it all wrong. I made it more painful than it had to be.

However, I was determined to nurse my child because I had read several books which discussed the benefits of nursing for nursing mothers and their babies. I can't describe how wonderful it feels to develop such a special bond with your child fostered through nursing. There has always been a gleam of trust and serenity in the eyes of my children whenever we shared what seemed to be endless gazes at one another while we nursed. I am so glad that I decided to go through with the nursing process. It has been a rewarding experience which has benefited both my children and myself immensely.

Lorinda: I wasn't able to breastfeed my first son as long as I would have liked to. Breastfeeding went smoothly while we were still in the hospital. However, after being home for a while, we started to have problems.

My son stopped nursing on one side. I quickly became engorged and, to make matters worse, I was not managing the pain well from my c-section operation. The only support person I knew of was one of the nursery nurses at the hospital. She had been very helpful and patient while my baby and I adjusted to nursing. I called her several times and again she was very patient.

She had given me several suggestions, such as trying different positions, expressing milk so as not to become too engorged, etc. She even suggested that I obtain a different breast pump (I was using, not very successfully, a manual cylindrical pump). She finally recommended that I contact La Leche for support. By that time I was already supplementing nursing with formula and I reluctantly decided to switch completely to formula.

While I was pregnant with my second son, I met a friend who happened to be a lactation consultant. I asked her if she would help me if I had problems nursing again. After the baby was born, her support was immeasurable. She allowed me to rent an electric breast pump (which was very easy to use) and she visited us on several occasions. Everything worked out well this time around as I nursed my son.

Colostrum

Lorinda: I was told that I wouldn't have milk immediately, but instead there would be colostrum which is really important to the baby. That is why I really wanted to breastfeed at the beginning, so if for some reason everything didn't work out with breasfeeding I would've already at least given the baby the benefit of colostrum.

While the baby was getting the colostrum it seemed like nothing was coming out and that made me a little anxious at first. But the nursery nurses were saying that, "You know, he is getting it," and I would say, "I can't see it." They would assure

❁ **DEFINITION:**
Colostrum is described as pre-milk, a high protein, high calorie fluid produced for a period of time before a woman actually produces breastmilk. Colostrum is the first nourishment the newborn baby who is breastfed will have. Though this fluid is almost transparent and sometimes very difficult for the new mother to see, it is there.

Colostrum contains the beginnings of the baby's immunologic protection, as well as nutrients, and is an important part of breastfeeding. In addition, it aids in the baby's elimination of meconium.

me that it was there though and I could see something clear, but it didn't seem like there was enough. But, of course, they reassured me and my pediatrician assured that it was very important that the baby get the colostrum even though it may not seem like it is enough.

Zaakira: I was so afraid. With my first child I was really scared and worried because I really didn't know how the process would work. You know, things like how long it would take for the milk to come in and I had so many negative people around me that didn't want me to breastfeed anyway. And my mother-in-law was like, "You better get some Similac. You better get it, the baby's hungry." Then, it was painful and I was thinking that I didn't want to do this anymore, it hurts. It was almost like I was intentionally putting my breast in the mouth of a lion or something.

And my mother-in-law, who was with me the whole time said, "Well you better do it, she's hungry," and I just wanted to cry. It did appear to me she was hungry and the milk wasn't there, it was just colostrum, which you can barely even see. I didn't give up though, I stuck it out. I did do something. I got some water – the glucose water they give you and I gave her some because I was so scared that she wasn't getting enough. I didn't want her to get dehydrated or anything, because even when you start nursing you don't know how much milk you're producing. You really don't know until you start seeing the milk and you're on an actual feeding schedule.

So, I was very worried about it. It took me about three weeks to get the whole nursing process under control and I'm so glad I stuck it out. With all of the negativity around me and the pain that went along with it and not knowing whether the child is getting enough; those are three components that would make anyone a little leary of breastfeeding. But, after having gone through it I realized that it would take a little while and then it would be fine.

For my other two children, I didn't worry about it at all. In fact, it seemed like for them the milk came in a lot faster and I don't know if it was because my body was accustomed to having produced milk before or what. Both of my other children also seemed to latch on better and I think it just came with the experience of knowing what to expect. I'm not sure whether there was a real difference, but in my mind there was a psychological difference because I had a new level of confidence. Anybody could say anything negative to me at that time and I was like, "Yeah right."

Elisa: Colostrum was definitely a big source of anxiety and stress. With my first child, since I couldn't see it, I was really afraid that she wasn't getting enough. She wouldn't suck very long. She would latch on and suck a few times and fall right to sleep everytime she got close to me. And I don't know if it was because I was warm or she was tired or she just got comfortable. We did everything we could to wake her up. We would touch her, move her around, undress her, talk to her, turn the lights on bright and she didn't care. She just fell asleep no matter what we did.

So, that's when I really felt that she definitely wasn't getting enough and she wasn't suckling enough for me to start producing milk. Needless to say, I was very paranoid about whether this colostrum was enough. And there was a little nurse's assistant from the islands who I treasure to this day because when she came in the baby had been sleeping for hours. I was so worried because we tried to wake her up every couple of hours and feed her, but she would fall right back to sleep. The woman said, "That baby needs some nourishment or she's just going to pass right away." And I was so upset, but my mother got a little medicine cup and started cup feeding the baby, first with a little sugar water and then formula.

My newborn daughter instantly came directly to life and was looking around, smiling and cooing. She hasn't slowed down yet. So, my fear that colostrum was not enough was bonafide, I think, because she wasn't suckling enough to give herself any energy. We ended up cup feeding her while in the hospital until my milk came in when we were at home.

With my second child, since I knew more about colostrum and I felt more confident in my breastfeeding ability having nursed my first for a year, I was alot more confident in the breastfeeding process. And, about 4 days before my son was born my husband was working in his office and I was watching television, when I felt my milk come in. I was used to that feeling because my children were so close together and I nursed my daughter until she was 11 months, which made me about 6 months pregnant with my second child.

It hadn't been that long since my milk production had stopped, so I was very used to the feeling of milk letting down. I thought it was really wierd, so I went into my husband's office and told him my milk had come in. He of course said, "Yeah, okay," as though I were crazy and I said, "No, it really has come in." So, I took my shirt off and tried to express some milk. Sure enough, out came colostrum! My husband said, "Well, I guess I better go pack my bag because the baby will be here any day now." He stopped his work and went upstairs to pack his over-night bag just in case I went into labor that night.

Once my son was born, he latched on very quickly the first time I tried to nurse him and has been eating beautifully since then. I think a lot of that has to do with the fact that I knew what I was doing. This time I didn't have to fumble or guess, I knew what I was doing and it was easier for both of us. I still did cup feed him a little in the hospital, supplementing him with formula because he was so heavy. He was almost 10 pounds and I was concerned about not making enough colostrum to keep up his body weight.

Michelle: I didn't have any anxieties about whether or not my baby was getting enough with colostrum, but people gave me anxieties. Newborns cry a lot and my mother-in-law kept saying, "He's probably not getting enough, he's not getting enough." And, she constantly asked me if my milk was in yet. I wasn't concerned about it initially, but she kind of made it a concern for me.

The nurses were very reassuring. They said that the baby was getting everything he needed with the colostrum. With Blake, my second child, for the first 24 hours after birth he slept continuously. And the nurse said that after birth they generally have enough food within them to carry them for the first 48 hours. With Quinn, my first baby, it took about 5 days for my milk to come in. With Blake it took about 2 days.

I had done enough reading to realize the beneficial effects of colostrum and knew that it was a part of the whole process that was needed. So, I didn't have anxieties, except that people tended to make me have them by the questions they would ask and some of the pressure they put on me. I would gain reassurance from the nurses or call the pediatrician and they would tell me to just block out what everyone else was saying.

More Information Please!

Elisa: I again feel that there was just not enough time spent in the childbirth preparation classes on breastfeeding. They got you through labor as though that was the hardest part of having children. The hardest part is when you take them home, but I just felt dumped because they didn't prepare you well at all for the whole breastfeeding experience.

Lorinda: There isn't enough information on breastfeeding, as far as the fact that there might be some problems and what you should do when those problems arise. I think that

❀

BREASTFEEDING BASICS: *Though breastfeeding is a natural process, it does require some practice on behalf of mom and baby, as well as some education on mom's part. The fact that breastfeeding is a natural physiological function has often resulted in mothers anxious to breastfeed getting hit with the reality that it takes work and commitment. They have been left out to dry, with everyone assuming that because they have breasts they will know what to do.*

1) Your colostrum will be the first nourishment the baby receives and is very good for baby, despite the fact that it can be difficult to see.

2) On occasion, larger newborns may need some supplementing with formula until your milk comes in. Let your baby guide you on this one, not the anti-breastfeeding relative. You'll soon discover the difference between baby's hungry nursing and the "I need to be comforted" nursing. If your baby is still frantically rooting after nursing on your colostrum for long periods, don't panic. You might try a little formula out of a small medicine cup. Your nurses in the hospital nursery can show you how this is done.

3) Your milk will come in 2-6 days after delivery.

4) When let-down occurs, you will know. You will be able to physically feel your milk coming into your breasts and often at this time will become engorged.

5) A lactation consultant can be a lifesaver for the mother and baby who are struggling. Some hospitals have them visit you after your child has been delivered, but you may have to request one. If you want to speak to someone in advance, ask your childbirth educator or call the La Leche League.

6) Be patient. Breastfeeding is not automatic for all moms and their newborns.

7) Take care of your nipples. Lansinoh® is a natural cream specifically for breastfeeding mothers. It is used to soften and protect against cracked nipples during breastfeeding or prenatally to prepare the nipple for breastfeeding and proactively prevent dryness, cracking or soarness.

8) When baby stops feeding, sometimes, especially with newborns, it is because baby needs to burp. Burp baby often and for as long as necessary initially. This will payoff in the long run with a baby who knows how to burp on its own.

(continued on page 173)

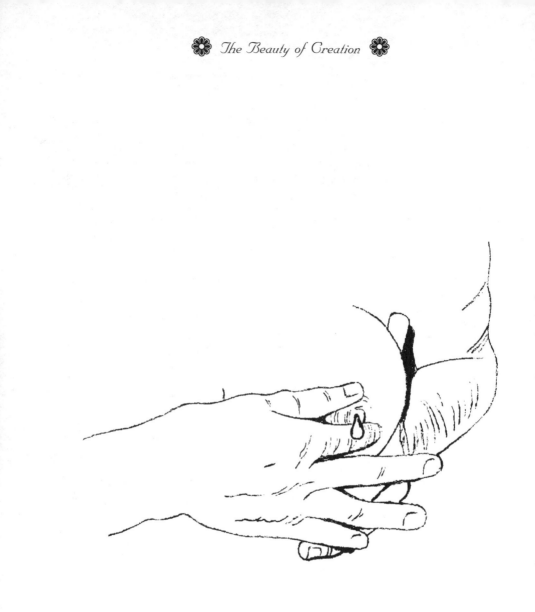

EXPRESSING MILK
(SEE EXPLANATION ON NEXT PAGE)

(continued from page 171)

9) *Your diet affects your breast milk. Onions, spicy foods and other strong tastes may turn baby off or give baby one heck of a case of gas. Your baby is eating what you eat.*

10) *Drugs, including liquor, will show up in your breast milk. For baby's sake, think about this while you are breastfeeding. If you must take prescripton medication, make sure your physician knows that you are breastfeeding and if there is any question ask your pediatrician.*

11) *Nutritionally speaking, your breast milk has all your baby's needs and is sufficient by itself for the first year and beyond, if this is a choice of yours. Though many choose to feed their baby's solid food very early, it is not an absolute necessity, but it can ease the demand on mommy.*

❀

EXPRESSING MILK:
Cupping the breast with your hand, place your thumb above the nipple and your forefinger below it at the beginning of the areola. Simply squeeze the thumb and forefinger together, and with practice comes the milk..

12) *When your breasts are full and for some reason baby isn't hungry, <u>expressing</u> milk or using a breast pump can help you avoid engorgement.*

13) *Your milk is liquid gold! If you are pumping milk, it can be stored in the refrigerator for about 48 hours and as many as 3 months or so in the freezer. This can be ideal for times when mommy is away or when daddy or other people are feeding baby with a bottle.*

14) *Don't defrost frozen milk and re-freeze or refrigerate it. Once it's thawed, baby either drinks it or it is gone.*

15) *Nursing mothers need plenty of fluids.*

16) *Though nursing is often seen as a contraceptive, you can get pregnant again while you are nursing!*

17) *Breastfeeding is not effortless and may sap some of your energy. If both you and your spouse understand this, it makes things easier.*

These are just some tips that might help a breastfeeding mother along the way. There is much more to it, however. Don't stop here.

needs to be emphasized more. Also, it needs to be made known that there is support and you should probably seek support before you deliver so that you can have it in place right when the baby is born.

Zaakira: I really think breastfeeding did increase my appetite initially. And then after I got accustomed to it I think that I just kept eating. I don't think I was supposed to.

I do really know that breastfeeding seriously impacted my appetite for the first 3 months and I was really getting hungry. Little babies can only drink so much and so they nurse for a little bit and they finish and then they come back every half hour to 45 minutes. I think that part is draining.

Once they get older and they know how to consume the milk and get a full feeding without falling asleep in between feeding from both sides, I think that it was less draining because it was not as frequent. With them being little, it was every 30 minutes, every 45 minutes and I was exhausted. I was tired, sleepy and I wanted to just be able to take a shower and do something for myself, but that seemed impossible. It seemed that every time I would think it was a free moment the baby would be hungry.

So I think that it's in the initial stages when it's more draining and you get hungrier because the baby's eating patterns are different because they're so young.

❀

Breastfeeding can be a wonderful time for baby and mom.
Good Luck!

Chapter 12
Hospital Eutopia

Elisa: With my first child I thought, while in the hospital, that I must be the best parent in the world. I was thinking, 'This child eats, makes a poopy and then goes right to sleep. My goodness, this is going to be the easiest thing ever.' The reason was because in the hospital my babies slept and slept some more. It seems like the minute we got them home they just wanted to be awake constantly, during the night, during the day.

It was harder the first time because I was not used to sleep deprivation. At one point with our first child my husband and I were just delirious and were joking, saying that it was like we were in a sleep deprivation study. We hadn't slept in so long. I remember my father-in-law saying, "Why don't you two sleep in shifts?" And I would get so upset and I remember saying, "How am I going to sleep with my baby screaming?" There was no way I could go to sleep then, especially when you're not used to it. I guess now I could sleep because I'm used to children crying.

My second baby slept a lot more at home. I think it was because my time was so short with him, because of our older child, that he was kind of forced to go back to sleep. He would rest, wake-up, play and then put himself back to sleep.

Their poopies got stinkier once we got home too. In the hospital it didn't even stink. You had to watch for them making their poopies. At home it would permeate the whole house it seemed. The diaper genie was on overtime trying to keep up with the output.

Lorinda: There was definitely a difference in the transition from being in the hospital after my children were born to being at home. In the hospital I really felt pampered. I mean you really don't have to do much. They bring the baby to you and you nurse him. And when the baby is asleep they take him to the nursery.

Some women told me from their experiences to let the baby go to the nursery and rest. They let the baby stay in your room if you request it. But I had gotten this advice from friends who said just let them take care of the baby in the nursery because you'll have plenty of time to do that.

Especially after my first child with the c-section, I was in some pain, so I took every advantage of the pampering they offered. And I really did feel pampered. In the hospital I had my meals prepared and everything. It was really good except for all of the times they come into your room to get different vital signs and other readings.

When I got home it was a different story, because basically I had to do everything with the help of my husband. We did everything by ourselves. So we were up a lot and I was trying to nurse which didn't go very well with the first child. It went well in the hospital, but not at home.

It was really a rude awakening with the first child. It was good though, or at least not bad, even though the first week was pretty rough. I was overwhelmed mostly not so much because of the care my son required, but because I wasn't successful breastfeeding and I was engorged without the support I needed. Also, because I was trying to breastfeed, I didn't take pain medicine for my c-section which meant that I was in pain a lot.

After I decided to put my first child on the bottle it was fine. We had visitors then and they just kind of took over. All I had to do for myself was eat. They were feeding him and changing him and bathing him. All I had to do was eat and take care of my pain.

My second child was smoother. Breastfeeding went well and we knew what to expect and what to prepare for.

Zaakira: With my first child, I kept her in the hospital room with me the whole time. I was exhausted by the time I got home. I didn't take advantage of using the nursery and getting some rest like I should have. I just kept the baby with me and I stayed up all night watching the baby because I was thinking, 'What if someone walks in while I'm sleeping and something happens to my baby.'

By the time I got home I was so exhausted already. So with my second and third child, when I felt very sleepy and I didn't think I could stay awake and be very attentive, I would call the nurse and have her come get the baby. And, of course, they would watch the baby in the nursery until I rested. If I had done that with my first child I would have felt so guilty about letting her go back to the nursery. But, after knowing that once you get home you are on your own, you've got to get some rest in the hospital.

My mother came and stayed with me for a week every time I had a child, but after she was gone it was just me. And I did find it very tiring. Once at home it did seem like the baby stayed awake more, because in the hospital if the baby was awake and I was sleepy, I would send her to the nursery and there would be someone taking care of her. I didn't have to worry about the baby's safety. But, when I was at home it was just me. If the baby was up, I was up.

Michelle: I think babies are their best in the hospital. In retrospect I think it's due to the fact that labor and delivery, or simply bringing a child into the world by whatever means, is stressful not only for the mother, but for the baby as well. Just like you need the recuperation time in the hospital, the baby needs it too. They are resting too, while in the hospital.

So, babies are usually at their best in the hospital. I can remember when we brought Quinn home, we thought it was a different baby. He was up constantly, had days and nights confused, was crying quite a bit, and it lasted probably 3 months. Blake slept continuously in the hospital. It was the same exact scenario. When we got him home he also had his days and nights confused, was sleeping no more than an hour at a time, was nursing constantly, and he leveled himself out at about 2 months.

The hospital baby is different from the baby that comes home, until that baby gets a little older and gets comfortable with nursing, etc. A lot of times they're pacifying themselves when they are nursing and not really eating or hungry. At first, and until they learn how to be productive eaters, they're getting used to their new environment. So, when they get home after resting in the hospital, they're just sometimes uncomfortable. I mean, think about it, they have been in a warm, dark place protected from everything and then all of a sudden they are out with all of this light and noise. So it takes some time to adjust.

Chapter 13
Tryin' Times, Cryin' Times

Ain't no need to worry, what the night is gonna bring
It'll be all over, in the morning

As wonderful as pregnancy and childbirth are, there are times that will test even the strongest of hearts. Sometimes the most difficult part of experiencing hard times is that you feel helpless and alone, even if you're surrounded by friends and family. Even during the beauty of creation there may be tears, sorrow, frustration and pain.

The good news is that you are not alone and some of the most difficult times produce the most wonderful outcomes. Take comfort and gain strength in our stories of trial and pain, realizing that it can work out all right and sometimes the only problem that exists is the fear and stress in your own mind.

In knowing of the experiences that other women have overcome, perhaps your cryin' and tryin' times won't be so bad afterall.

Zaakira: You can't even explain how it feels to find out that your child is ill or has a deformity. I was floored when they mentioned that my second child may have Down Syndrome. There was nothing to indicate that the pregnancy wasn't perfect and they just thrust this on us. It was very distressing.

On top of just getting this devastating news in a very nonchalant way, the process of finding out whether or not she had Down Syndrome was a 7 day process. They had to do all kinds of tests and wait for blood work to return from the lab. That 7 days was a living nightmare.

But with faith in the Creator and many long, heartfelt prayers, we were able to overcome this trial. When you are a parent, your child is so beautiful to you no matter what. We prayed for the best, but we prepared ourselves for the worst. We started finding out information about how to care for a child with Down Syndrome. We also found out what kind of learning disabilities our child might have. We even found the school in our area for students with Down Syndrome.

Ultimately, we knew that whatever the circumstances were, we loved our child. We intended to care for her the best way we could. Fortunately, we did not have to explore the options that we had considered before the results of her tests came back. Nefertari did not have Down Syndrome. We were so thankful to the Creator for having Blessed us with another healthy child!

Michelle: Throughout my first pregnancy there were several scary moments. However, the one in particular that comes to the forefront of my mind is this: I was approximately 11 weeks pregnant. My husband was downstairs preparing dinner and I was upstairs watering plants. Suddenly I felt as though I were bleeding. I rushed to the bathroom to find that I was in fact passing blood.

At that point I screamed hysterically for my husband and when he got upstairs and saw what was happening, he panicked! *He* was hysterical. I quickly determined that I had to calm myself and become strong for both of us. I instructed him to dial the doctor's emergency number (which was on speed dial). When he got through on the emergency line, another practice's physicians were on call. I was lying down and I could tell the doctor was asking Al a series of questions, because he was rambling and out of sorts. So I took the phone.

The doctor asked if I was cramping, if I had filled a pad with blood, and a number of other questions. When I responded "no" to his entire series of questions, he instructed me to lay down and come in first thing in the morning.

Dinner burned, while my husband sifted through the toilet and placed the material I had passed into a container. When we went in for the examination the next morning, he handed the container of bloody matter to the nurse. She looked at us and smiled, but the time leading up to that smile was extremely tough.

I was told there was a bruise in my uterus, which caused the passing of blood and was put on bed rest for 2 weeks.

During my next pregnancy, I started to spot. This time the spotting was a brownish color, and again, I was scared to death, especially since I was coming off of a recent miscarriage. However, I was placed on Progesterone for 12 weeks and it all stopped. As you can see, fears don't always have to mean tears.

Elisa: I had bleeding with my first child, Nandi, between 7 and 9 weeks. When I did start bleeding I fell on the floor and starting crying, saying "I just can't do this again," since I had just had a miscarriage at 11 weeks with the pregnancy prior to Nandi's. I beat myself up about it before I had been to the doctor, before I made a phone call, or before I even really knew what was going on.

I wish I could take back that time of letting myself think that I had somehow failed at mothering...again.

Lorinda: Right after my first son was born, coming home and him not being able to nurse, or me not having the support I needed as far as a lactation consultant, that was a crying time. With the hormones and the pain from my c-section, I cried a few days there. Just uncontrollable tears. I tried to stop them and I couldn't. I just couldn't stop them, but they didn't last thank God.

KEEP YOUR HEAD UP!

Chapter 14
Complications of
Pregnancy & Childbirth

Most pregnancies go without a hitch, or at least only minor problems when they do occur at all. However, sometimes complications do arise that are more than just hitches. Even so, most of them can be resolved uneventfully. There are a number of complications that can occur during pregnancy and others during childbirth. This chapter presents these complications for your general information.

We encourage you not to spend a lot of time and energy worrying about every little ache and pain, especially during your pregnancy. You will have those and they are quite natural. Enjoy your pregnancy to the fullest. If, however, you have any concerns and problems arise, consult your physician.

COMPLICATIONS OF PREGNANCY

Miscarriage - A miscarriage is the loss of a baby, which occurs naturally, before week 20 of pregnancy. A miscarriage is also referred to as a *spontaneous abortion*.

When a miscarriage is occurring or likely to occur, the mother-to-be usually has spotting or bright red bleeding in significant amounts. (Spotting can occur in most pregnancies and is not necessarily a sign that anything is wrong. Don't panic, notify your doctor.) Cramping of the uterus will also occur and, in conjunction with the bleeding and vaginal discharge, will become more severe.

On physical examination, if the cervix is dilated it is assumed that the miscarriage is taking place or has taken place. Nothing can be done at this point. In most cases the baby will have already died, causing the miscarriage.

If there is no dilatation and the baby is shown to be alive (through ultrasound), chances are good that the miscarriage will not progress and baby will be fine. Bed rest and a cessation of intercourse and other activities may be recommended depending on the circumstances.

If the miscarriage progresses, the baby may be lost and expelled from the uterus (clots and tissue will be expelled, either partially or completely, emptying the contents of the uterus.)

When a miscarriage results in the contents of the uterus being partially expelled, it is called an *incomplete abortion*. A D and C (dilation and curettage) will remove the remaining fetal tissue from the uterus. This procedure is usually performed at the hospital.

Stillbirth is the term used to describe the loss of a baby after the 20th week.

After a miscarriage or a stillbirth, two very important things must occur. The physician must attempt to determine the cause and the mother who has suffered this loss, must have support to deal with it. There are resources that your nurse or physician can share with you for coping with miscarriage and still-birth.

The loss of your baby should not be "blown off" or treated as though it were supposed to happen. It can be a traumatic experience and needs to be recognized.

Anemias - These are conditions marked by an abnormally low red blood cell count or an insufficient amount of hemoglobin (which carries blood oxygen). Iron deficiency is the most common type of anemia. It can be treated with Iron tablets. Sometimes folic acid deficiency also occurs, which can be treated with folate tablets.

* *Sickle cell anemia* is a disease that can be inherited and results in the red blood cells containing an abnormal form of hemoglobin, which results in a reduced amount of oxygen and crescent or sickle-shaped cells. These sickle-shaped cells also can block smaller blood vessels and break up, damaging these vessels and causing reduced oxygen supply to major organs. The disease affects African

Americans predominantly, in the United States.

In pregnant women with sickle-cell anemia, infections can occur more frequently. Urinary tract infections (UTI's) and uterine infections are most common. High blood pressure and other complications can occur in pregnant women with sickle-cell. If you have sickle-cell anemia, consult your specialist and your obstetrician about pregnancy risks.

Ectopic Pregnancy - This is when the pregnancy implants and begins its development outside of the uterus. It happens most commonly in the fallopian tube. Other locations of ectopic pregnancy include the cervix, ovary and abdomen.

Symptoms of an ectopic pregnancy can include spotting or light bleeding, cramps, pain and tenderness on one side, pressure in the rectal area from accumulating blood (which may result from tearing of the fallopian tube wall as the baby grows), etc. If the fallopian tube ruptures, this may cause tremendous blood loss and more severe symptoms, including shock and sharp pain.

Early diagnosis presents the best opportunity for resolution without severe damage to the mother. Baby will not survive an ectopic pregnancy. However, treatment can prevent damage to mom.

Your doctor will diagnose an ectopic pregnancy based upon several signs and your symptoms. For example, if your tests show that you are pregnant, yet the size of your uterus is small for the number of weeks of the pregnancy, this may lead the doctor to suspect ectopic pregnancy. Further, if upon ultrasound the uterus is empty or there is blood in the abdominal or pelvic cavity, the doctor's suspicions have moved closer to being confirmed.

The doctor can look directly at the pregnancy using an instrument called a laparoscope that is inserted through a small incision in the abdomen.

The pregnancy is then either removed surgically or using the drug, methotrexate.

Hyperemesis gravidarum - This is extreme or excessive vomiting. In this condition, usually morning sickness is replaced by a much more severe and frequent vomiting.

Sometimes hospitalization is required to replace fluids via an I.V. and control dehydration. Antiemetics (anti-vomiting drugs) can also be given. At such time that vomiting and dehydration are controlled, mom can start eating bland foods and increase her intake as she is able. Vomiting usually stops within a few days.

Rh Incompatibility - The Rh blood group (molecules on the surface of the red blood cell) of the mother and baby are in conflict. An Rh negative mother may develop antibodies against the red blood cells of an Rh positive baby. This is rarely a problem in first pregnancies. If detected, your doctor can discuss treatment options with you.

Placenta Previa - This is when the placenta implants over, or partially over, the cervix. Vaginal bleeding without pain can become significant late in pregnancy and the blood may be bright red. An ultrasound helps your doctor make a definitive diagnosis.

A c-section is usually the course of action once the baby is far enough along. Other options range from bed rest to transfusion, depending on the amount of blood loss.

Abruptio Placenta - The placenta detaches from the uterus before childbirth, either incompletely or completely.

Sometimes bleeding can be seen externally and in other cases blood is trapped behind the displaced placenta. The reduction of oxygen supply to the baby depends on the degree to which the placenta has detached, as does the severity of symptoms mom will feel.

Hospitalization is the course of action after diagnosis and treatment can range from bed rest to cesarean.

Preeclampsia - This is high blood pressure experienced during pregnancy. It can develop between the 20th week and one week after delivery. It can be accompanied by retention of fluid, which causes swelling, or by protein in the urine.

Eclampsia is a more severe form of preeclampsia in which siezures and/or a coma could result. Symptoms include swelling in the face and hands, with excessive weight gain from the retained water.

As the condition worsens it can result in blurred vision, irritation, insufficient urine production, headaches, abdominal pain, etc.

If preeclampsia goes untreated, eclampsia can result.

Bed rest can be important and sometimes hospitalization is required when mild preeclampsia doesn't improve. If hospitalization does help, the baby must be delivered as soon as possible.

With severe preeclampsia, hospitalization and bed rest are immediate. Treatment with I.V. medication and fluids is usually effective in relieving symptoms and reducing blood pressure. The baby can be delivered safely once the blood pressure is under control.

When a complication called HELLP syndrome arises from severe preeclampsia or eclampsia, this can mean problems for the mother-to-be. It involves the breakdown of red blood cells (**Hemolysis**), Liver damage (detected by **E**levated **L**iver enzymes), and impaired blood clotting (indicated by a **L**ow **P**latelet count).

Gestational Diabetes - This is diabetes that begins or is first noticed during pregnancy. Pregnancy produces changes in the body that sometimes can result in an increased demand for insulin and sometimes in insulin resistance. This presents a problem in handling the increased blood sugar that pregnancy brings.

Urticaria - This is a common rash seen in pregnant women that may arise any time after the 24th week of pregnancy, but usually toward the end of pregnancy. It causes a sometimes hive-like patchy, itchy abdominal area and can spread to other areas, such as the thighs, buttocks, etc. The rash

usually lasts only 2 to 4 days when treated. Treatment usually consists of corticosteroid cream.

Trophoblastic Disease - A hydatidiform mole often results in a uterus that increases in size too fast to be in proportion with the progress of the pregnancy. A trophoblast is the group of cells that line the amniotic sac and form villi to assist in implantation. In this disease, these trophoblastic cells fail to assist in the formation of a viable placenta. Instead, these cells form a proliferated mass, called a hydatidiform mole. It is rare.

In addition to the quickly growing uterus, women may experience bleeding, no baby movement, the absence of a heartbeat and severe vomiting and nausea.

Once the diagnosis is made, the remaining contents of the uterus must be cleared, just as in a miscarriage. Because this "molar pregnancy" is proliferative, follow up is necessary and another D and C may need to be performed to remove any additional material that has grown. Follow-up is very key since there is the outside chance of the molar pregnancy developing into *metastic trophoblastic disease*, which means the mole is now malignant and forms a *choriocarcinoma* (cancer).

❀

COMPLICATIONS OF CHILDBIRTH

Premature Labor - This is the beginning of labor before the 37th week of pregnancy. It is marked by the early effacement and dilatation of the cervix. When premature labor is associated with the rupture of membranes or vaginal bleeding, it won't be stopped. When the labor is not associated with bleeding or rupture of membrane, bed rest and liquids may help stop labor.

The problems with the baby being born before the 37th week include underdeveloped respiratory and immune systems, among other things.

Premature Rupture of Membranes - This is defined as any instance when the membranes rupture, or the water breaks, more than one hour before labor begins. In a mother who has carried her baby to term, labor will be induced in this case.

Hypotonic Uterine Dysfunction - This is when a patient's labor fails to progress past the pre or early labor phase, with less than 4cm dilatation, irreglar contractions and little effacement.

Pitocin stimulation is often used to advance labor.

Hypertonic Uterine Dysfunction - This type of dysfunction causes contractions to be too strong and too close together during labor. If Pitocin is being used it should be discontinued and pain medication can be given to the pregnant mother. Other medications that slow the progression of labor might also be considered.

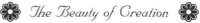

Amniotic Fluid Embolism - This is another very rare occurrence in which amniotic fluid gets into the pulmonary circulation of the pregnant mother. It can potentially cause shock, dangerously increased heart rate, heart irregularity, cardiac arrest and death.

Umbilical Cord Prolapse - This rare situation is marked by the umbilical cord presenting ahead of the baby. It can be *occult* prolapse (when membranes haven't yet ruptured) or *overt* (membranes have already ruptured).

Breech presentation is the most common time that this occurs. This situation is treated by immediate delivery of the baby by cesarean, to prevent oxygen reduction due to compression of the cord.

Abnormal Fetal Presentation - The different abnormal presentations are 1) *complete breech* presentation is when baby's bottom is down, but baby's knees are bent almost as if it were sitting buddha style; 2) *frank breech* presentation, in which the baby's bottom is down toward the cervix, the hips are flexed, but the knees are straight with the feet up around the baby's head area.

NORMAL PRESENTATION

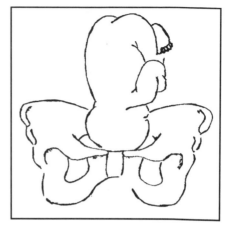

COMPLETE BREECH PRESENTATION

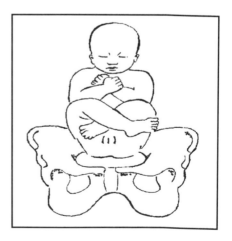

FRANK BREECH PRESENTATION

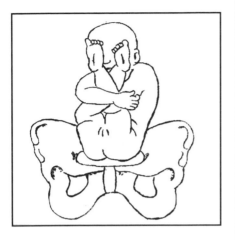

3) *Face* presentation is when the baby's head is facing toward the cervix, but instead of being down, the face is looking toward the cervix and vagina. Vaginal delivery is not an option here; 4) *brow* presentation is similar to face, except the head is not hyperextended so that the face is looking down. Instead, the brow, or forehead, presents first. Vaginal delivery is not an option; 5) *footling* presentation is when one or both legs are the first thing to present. It's almost as if the baby is stepping out of the womb. In many of these cases an emergency c-section may be necessary once the abnormal presentation is discovered (if not previously known) in order to prevent brain or nerve damage to the baby.

Shoulder Dystocia - A rare complication in which one of the baby's shoulders gets stuck in the birth canal, unable to pass the mother's pelvic bone. The obstetrician may try a variety of physical manipulations of both the mother and baby. On occasion the baby's shoulder bone is broken in the process.

Fetal Distress - This is a broad term used to describe a baby who is in trouble during the childbirth process. It is most commonly due to a reduction in oxygen supply. There are a number of potential causes, including the cord being around the baby's neck, compression of the cord with cord proplapse, etc.

A fetal monitor will keep the doctor aware of the baby's condition and when necessary an emergency c-section is performed.

Uterine Hemorrhage PostPartum - Excessive blood loss after the delivery of the baby. It can be due to a part of the placenta remaining in the uterus or the failure of the uterus to contract to help close the open vessels left by the detachment of the placenta.

A certain amount of blood loss is normal during and after delivery.

These are some of the potential problems that occur during pregnancy and childbirth. Most of them are rare and your pregnancy will probably progress just fine. Your doctor will be able to give more complete answers to any questions you may have. Never hesitate to ask, but at the same time, don't spend all of your pregnancy worrying about what could go wrong!

Enjoy yourself! You are participating in a wonderful miracle. It is the beauty of creation!

The following chapter by Dr. Anne Graham, dealing with high-risk pregnancy, is also very informative regarding complications. And finally, if you like, you can also go back and read some of the more positive and uplifting information in this book. It might take your mind off of complications. Good luck! We know you will do well.

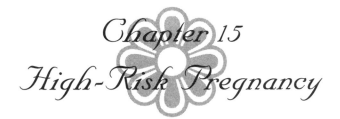

Chapter 15
High-Risk Pregnancy

Dr. Anne Graham

Thank goodness that a lot of patients now prepare for pregnancy by doing their research prior to getting pregnant and attempting to conceive in the best possible circumstances. However, most patients find themselves pregnant without consciously planning a pregnancy, and find out at a time when most fetal organs have formed. The best advice for patients contemplating pregnancy is to plan your pregnancy, that is make a conscious effort to find out more about the process; about conceiving and how your pregnancy might be affected by both lifestyle and any disease process you might have.

Although most pregnancies are uncomplicated, approximately 20-30% of women will develop complications during the course of their pregnancy or during the process of labor and delivery. Patients and their physicians must remain vigilant throughout their pregnancy to be sure that complications, if they do arise, are diagnosed early to allow prompt therapy and/or measures to be taken in order to lessen the risk of a poor outcome.

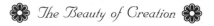
What is a High–Risk Pregnancy?

Any condition that may place the mother or her baby at risk for a negative pregnancy experience is, by definition, high risk. In some cases, these conditions exist prior to pregnancy, but often complications develop during pregnancy that put either the mother or baby at risk. These pregnancies are considered to be high risk. During pregnancy, a woman's body undergoes significant alterations so that a disease process that was well controlled prior to pregnancy, could possibly be not as well controlled during the pregnancy and may have an impact such that the mother is at increased risk. For these patients, it is important that prior to conceiving they visit a physician, one who is well versed in high-risk obstetrics and capable of developing a plan of care that will not only decrease risk prior to conception, but optimize both maternal and fetal well being. This is referred to as preconceptual counseling or prepregnancy planning.

What Can a Patient Do In Order to Optimize a Healthy Outcome for Both Her and Her Baby?

Mothers as well as fathers can impact the development of their fetus by ensuring that they provide a healthy environment in which to conceive. Whereas the impact of maternal diseases on conception and fetal development has been well defined, the effect of male disease on pregnancy is yet to be determined. For example, pregnant women who have diabetes prior to pregnancy increase their risk for fetal birth defects or miscarriages if their blood sugars are poorly controlled around the time of conception. However, this risk is lessened as blood glucose is brought under control.

Also, women who have high blood pressure may benefit from switching to similarly effective medication that does not increase the chance of causing birth defects in the fetus. It is important that all women who have a chronic condition consult with their obstetrician, or the physician treating the condition, prior to conceiving, in order to determine what preparations one must make to achieve the best possible outcome for mother and baby.

Diabetes and Pregnancy

Diabetes is an endocrine disorder in which insufficient insulin is produced by the body. As a result, blood glucose levels rise. Diabetes can be classified into pregestational diabetes and gestational diabetes. Pregestational diabetes is further classified according to non-insulin dependent diabetes mellitus, NIDDM (Type 1), or insulin dependent diabetes mellitus, IDDM (Type 2). There are other classifications of diabetes made by many obstetricians/gynecologists that take into consideration how long-standing the disease is, as well as the age of the patient at onset. All women who have pregestational diabetes are high-risk. Mothers who develop diabetes during pregnancy are at high-risk both during their pregnancy and are at increased risk for diabetes during their lifetime.

Pregestational diabetes is associated with an increased risk for early miscarriages, increased chance for birth defects or malformations, and increased complications of pregnancy such as hypertension during pregnancy. This is true especia¹ y if the disease affects organs such as the eyes or kidneys. These women must therefore plan their pregnancies very carefully and at the times when their diabetes is under great control.

During the pregnancy, patients must monitor their blood sugars frequently in order to maintain a normal blood sugar range. A normal range appears to be associated with better outcome for both the baby and mother. The diabetic mother is also at increased risk for birth defects such as heart defects and the fetus must have a special ultrasound in order to be able to detect these abnormalities should they occur.

Because of extra glucose and other growth factors, the fetuses are at increased risk for macrosomic growth (larger than normal), due to several growth factors associated with diabetes and insulin, and this may increase the chances of having a cesarean section.

Even with gestational diabetes alone, the risk of a large infant is also greater when compared to mothers who have a normal blood sugar test result. A special diet (offered by the ADA or American Diabetic Association) ensuring that glucose remains normal throughout pregnancy may decrease this risk.

Hypertension and Pregnancy

Many women have elevated blood pressure (chronic hypertension) prior to pregnancy. High blood pressure that develops during pregnancy is called by a number of names including gestational hypertension or, if it is accompanied by other factors such as kidney involvement and edema (swelling), it is called preeclampsia. Preeclampsia is fairly common in first time mothers and usually occurs towards the end of pregnancy. Most pregnant women will have some swelling during pregnancy, especially in the latter months and in hot weather. This does not necessarily mean that they have preeclampsia.

Chronic hypertension places the patient at high-risk and the outcome is determined by (1) the cause of the underlying hypertension, (2) the involvement of the kidneys and other organs (i.e. heart), which can be damaged by the elevated blood pressure. Some anti-hypertensive medications may be taken during pregnancy. The patient should be able to monitor her blood pressure at home and should be on a regimen of anti-hypertensive medication that will not harm her baby. Mothers on medications that increase the risk for the fetus and cause congenital birth defects can be switched to another drug that is considered safe during pregnancy.

Chronic hypertension is associated with an increased risk for complications such as low birth weight babies, intrauterine growth restriction (IUGR), increased risk for placental separation (placenta abruptio) and risk for preeclampsia. If the condition of preeclampsia deteriorates even further, eclampsia develops. This is where the disease has progressed sufficiently to bring on convulsions.

For most patients, preeclampsia cannot be detected except during regular check-ups when blood pressure begins to go up. This blood pressure increase may not be accompanied by a significant change in the mothers feeling of well being. Usually some swelling develops and protein spills into the urine. Depending on the physician, a number of remedies, including bed rest or anti-hypertensive medication can be indicated to prolong the pregnancy to the point that the fetus is able to be delivered.

Women with hypertension are also monitored with ultrasound to ensure that the baby is growing adequately, since high blood pressure may be associated with damage to the placenta and the development of growth restriction (size smaller than average). This is especially common if the hypertension is not well controlled. As most preeclampsia develops after the 20th week of pregnancy, it is important that the patient be seen frequently for the physician to make the diagnosis.

Although increase in blood pressure may be the first sign of preeclampsia, usually chronic headaches, visual changes or pain in the right upper abdomen are significant indicators of worsening condition. This pain is sometimes confused with indigestion and may require treatment usually involving antihypertensive medication, bed rest and, in some cases, delivery.

What You Can Do

A number of lifestyle changes can be undertaken which may modify high blood pressure:

- ✿ increasing the calcium in your diet
- ✿ resting for a few hours each day
- ✿ taking your blood pressure at home to be aware of factors that cause it to go up and modify these situations.

Preterm Labor and Premature Rupture of Membranes

Approximately 7% of women end up delivering prior to 37 weeks, making their babies premature. Full term is considered to be at 37-42 weeks of gestation. Prematurity is a major risk factor for poor outcome in these fetuses and contributes to 80% of the complications seen in all newborns. The younger the gestational age at delivery, the more likely it is to cause long term complications resulting from prematurity. These long-term complications may include chronic lung disease, brain hemorrhage and eye damage because of the use of oxygen therapy needed to keep the baby alive. Premature babies lungs are not quite ready to breathe air, so they cannot get sufficient oxygen. In addition, blood vessels in the brain are more fragile making them more likely to bleed.

How Do You Know If You Are At Risk?

Most preterm deliveries occur with patients who do not have a risk factor for preterm labor, making it very difficult to intervene in time to stop delivery. Preterm labor can be treated by a number of drugs provided that it is recognized promptly. Therapy is initiated to prevent the cervix from changing or opening up. As with most diseases, the earlier the intervention, the greater the chance of successfully keeping the pregnancy until such time that the baby is able to survive outside of the uterus with the least amount of complications.

Most patients have uterine contractions throughout pregnancy. With the use of sensitive instrumentation, one can measure these small contractions. The difficulty arises in attempting to decide which contractions are the real ones that cause cervical change and which are simply ineffective contractures.

Most of the time, this is very difficult to determine. Physicians are left to assess the cervix in order to see if there are any cervical changes. As in all diseases, the best monitoring methodology for preterm labor is you the patient. Therefore, all patients should be educated regarding the warning signs and symptoms of preterm labor so that they can report them promptly to their physician.

What Places You At High–Risk of Preterm Labor?

Although preterm labor occurs most in women who do

not have a risk factor, there are some known factors that may place you at increased risk. These conditions may include having more than one fetus in utero, such as twins or triplets; having an incompetent cervix (a weak cervix); uterine malformations where the uterus is known to be deformed; vaginal infections with so called nonspecific vaginitis or bacterial vaginosis; abnormalities of the fetus; bleeding; and physical trauma.

In addition, some other conditions that are associated with preterm labor include previous preterm labor or delivery, which increases risk approximately two and a half times; and previous lacerations of the cervix or trauma to the cervix especially during previous deliveries and/or uterine surgery.

Warning signs of preterm labor include:

(1)   Uterine contractions. This is where your uterus begins to tighten and the sensation spreads over all of your uterus. This may last for about 20 seconds, at a rate usually of 4 an hour, for more than 1 to 2 hours.

(2)   Menstrual-type cramps.

(3)   Dull pain in the lower back, either constant or rhythmic, not relieved by changing position. This is not the same pain that women get from carrying their babies late in pregnancies.

(4)   Persistent diarrhea.

(5)   Crampy intestinal pain.

(6)   Vaginal discharge greater than normal, especially if it tends to be very mucousy or if it is tinged with blood.

(7)   General feeling that something is wrong.

(8)   Lower pelvic pressure as opposed to lower abdominal pain or pressure in the front due to the weight of the baby.

If the situation is not preterm labor, these symptoms should usually go away with lying down and drinking lots of fluids. If this does not stop your feeling of contractions, then it is important to notify your physician immediately. Most patients do not like to call their physicians, especially at night, but the fact is that most physicians would rather intervene early and prevent preterm labor. Additionally, most women can be evaluated in the hospital, if not during office hours.

Since uterine contractions that cause cervical change (preterm labor) versus those that do not (Braxton-Hicks), cannot be differentiated on history alone, we think that most regular contractions should be evaluated in order to prevent preterm labor. The most common type of cervical evaluation is a digital examination. It is an examination done through the vagina in order to assess the cervix. However, with the advent of ultrasound, transvaginal ultrasound is used now to assess both the length of the cervix (effacement) and whether or not the cervix is opening from the top like a funnel, called funneling. These may show early signs of a change indicative of preterm labor.

New tests are available that can predict which patients may be in preterm labor. These include the Sal Test, a saliva test that tests for a hormone estriol in the saliva. It increases when labor may occur in the following 2 to 3 weeks. Another test is called fetal fibronectin, a substance that is released from between the cervix and the membranes when changes occur within the cervix. These tests are easily performed and the results are usually available within 48 hours.

How Do We Treat Preterm Labor?

Preterm labor is treated by a number of medications. Sometimes the uterus is contracting simply because the patient is too active and this can easily be remedied by bed rest and increased fluid, which improves the blood supply to the uterus. Sufficient water throughout your pregnancy is important to maintain hydration and to decrease your risk for uterine contractions. In addition, a sensible awareness regarding your pregnancy, considering what is normal versus what is abnormal, is important for the diagnosis of preterm labor in order for early intervention to occur.

Treatment therapy involves a number of agents since therapy of preterm labor is an evolving field. All of the drugs used for the treatment of preterm labor are usually safe for you and your baby, although there are some possible risks. In addition, at times when there is the threat of preterm delivery, you may need steroid hormones to encourage your baby's lungs to develop more quickly.

The medications that are used for preterm labor include magnesium sulfate, usually given intravenously, and Terbutaline given by injection or orally. It is controversial whether or not it is an effective agent, however, the Terbutaline pump has been used successfully in treating a number of cases and is associated with less side effects than oral Terbutaline. Calcium channel blockers are medications mainly used for hypertension, however, they have also been used for preterm labor. Indomethacin, another drug, can be used intermittently throughout pregnancy to treat a number of conditions including preterm labor and extra fluid around the baby, called polyhdramnios.

Premature Rupture of Membranes

Preterm rupture of membranes is when your water breaks prior to 37 weeks. Most times premature rupture of membranes either causes contractions to occur or is the result of contractions. Premature rupture of membranes can be caused by preterm labor, infection of the bladder or uterus, incompetent cervix, poor strength of the membranes, family history of premature rupture and preterm labor.

Premature rupture of membranes can be associated with a number of complications. These include decreased amniotic fluid around your baby, called oligohydramnios, or infection.

If rupture of membranes occurs very early in pregnancy, it is serious and is usually associated with other complications. Amniotic fluid around the baby keeps it within an environment that decreases the risk of infection. It provides a means for the baby to turn and move freely, while protecting the umbilical cord, that is the cord that carries nutrients from the placenta to the baby. This allows the baby to grow and develop without any restriction of its movement or the breathing movement of its chestwall. Ruptured membranes and oligohydramnios, or decreased amniotic fluid, may be associated with a number of problems including compression of the umbilical cord restricting the blood flow to the baby. Early in pregnancy, it may also be associated with failure of development or restriction of the development of the fetal lungs (pulmonary hypoplasia) preventing the baby from breathing at the time of its birth. Intrauterine infection may also occur. Compression of the cord may cause a cord accident, causing the baby to die. Ruptured membranes and oligohydramnios have also been associated with an increased risk for placental separation.

Depending on the gestational age, therapy may include administration of steroids to hasten lung development and delivery or expectant management. Expectant management is simply observing the baby and evaluating the mother on a periodic basis for signs of infection and for fetal well being, while allowing the baby to continue its growth.

Some patients with ruptured membranes may actually have a high leak, that is a rupture that is not over the cervix. As a result, the leaking stops and the baby goes on to accumulate fluid. This decreases the risk of infection and poor prognosis associated with ruptured membranes and oligohydramnios.

Bleeding During Pregnancy

The initial reaction of any patient bleeding during pregnancy is, " I am going to lose my baby." Perhaps this is the most frightening experience that most patients can have. Bleeding during pregnancy should not be considered normal. In fact, most patients do not have bleeding, therefore, there should be a reason for the bleeding. However, as with all symptoms there are some causes that do not place you or your baby in danger and there are some that can serve as a warning sign that something serious is happening.

Bleeding can occur from a number of sources. Either from the cervix or the uterus. During pregnancy, the lining on the inside of the cervix called endocervical mucosa begins to migrate outwards over the mouth of the cervix. This endocervical mucosal lining has much more blood supply than the normal covering of the vagina and the cervix. As a result of that, it is more prone to bleeding if it is touched. Some patient's bleeding may occur as a result of disturbance of the mucosa, including vaginal sexual intercourse or constipation. If the bleeding is self-limiting and can usually be connected to some recent event such as having sex, it usually is not a problem. However, if there had been no causes of bleeding initially, then it may be of a more serious nature.

Some other causes of bleeding from the cervix may include a cervical polyp, which usually can be seen on evaluation with a vaginal scan. These are finger-like projections of tissue which have more blood supply and are more fragile, making them more likely to bleed. Most patients who bleed from these causes, however, usually have simply a pinkish tinge or spotting rather than frank bleeding. Bleeding like a period is a little bit more serious. Causes of this kind of bleeding may include changes in the cervix associated with incompetent or weak cervix, or may include bleeding from the placenta, especially if it is over the cervical opening as in placenta previa. In some cases, the placenta begins to separate and as a result of that blood accumulates inside of the uterus and then is passed through the cervix into the vagina. This places the pregnancy at increased risk and is a sign of threatened miscarriage. These pregnancies must be followed closely with ultrasound in order to document the size of the bleed if present within the uterus, and in order to ensure that the fetus continues to do well.

In later pregnancy if the placenta separates as in abruptio placenta, it can increase the risk to the pregnancy. In abruption, the placenta separates from the wall of the uterus and increases the risk to the baby since there is not sufficient placental blood flow to provide adequate nutrition and oxygen for the baby. Such pregnancies must be watched carefully to ensure that the baby continues to grow and to develop. It is also important to assess if there are reasons that may cause a placental separation including conditions such as smoking or hypertension.

Perhaps one of the most significant causes of spotting and/or bleeding during pregnancy is cervical change. This is the so-called "bloody show" that is seen in labor or at term. In early pregnancy or in the middle of pregnancy, if spotting is in association with uterine contractions, it may be indicative of either incompetent cervix or preterm labor. Therefore, if bleeding presents in association with uterine contractions, it is very important that you consult your physician in order to rule out threatened loss or preterm labor.

Certainly, bleeding which is a common occurrence during pregnancy is worrisome, but only signifies that further evaluation is needed. It increases the chance of something being wrong, but does not necessarily mean a loss of your pregnancy.

Mother You Are in Charge

A very important part of your role during either a low or

high-risk pregnancy is to ensure that you notify your physician if you are feeling different during your pregnancy. Although you are going to your physician in order for them to take care of you and your unborn child, it is important to realize that the time that your physician or your care provider spends observing your baby is very small compared to the amount of time that you are with your baby. Therefore, mothers should be the ultimate watchers to ensure that their pregnancy is going fine. It is important to educate yourself regarding your pregnancy, notice what is going on and what is normal for pregnancy, and especially what is normal for you and your baby.

Fetal movement, which most people begin to feel at approximately 18-24 weeks of pregnancy is one such normal event that you can monitor in order to ensure that your baby is happy.

The baby has a normal daily pattern of movement that is fairly unique for that baby. In fact, fetal movement counting is a means to assess fetal well being. Some babies move in the morning, some late at night, some after eating. However, on a daily basis the pattern should be approximately the same. Early in pregnancy this movement may be felt as vigorous kicks. Later on as there is less room for the baby, kicks are not felt as much and the baby wiggles or tries to turn. This can be used as a means to ensure fetal well being and that everything is going fine with your pregnancy. You should be encouraged to note any alterations in fetal movement to your physician as your pregnancy progresses. Some physicians will provide you with objective methods to document fetal movement in order to track how the pregnancy is doing. Remember, a decrease in fetal movement can potentially be an early warning sign that something is not going right with your pregnancy.

The Secret of a Successful High-Risk Pregnancy

Barring events over which we have no control, pregnancy should be a time for you to participate in the ongoing care and watchfulness under which your baby develops. The best patient is an informed and educated one. That is, informed regarding what the next sequence of events in her care is going to be and what developmental milestones are occurring in her fetus, so that she can relate the occurrence or nonoccurrence of these as her pregnancy progresses. Therefore, in selecting your care provider, it is important that there is a degree of trust and communication that will allow you to discuss any and all questions no matter how insignificant you may think that they are. Most physicians would prefer that a patient get information from them and would have patients relate happenings regarding their pregnancy at an early enough time so that they can take the necessary steps to make alterations in their care. For a successful pregnancy, it is important that this feeling of trust be incorporated for the best outcome for you and your baby.

For high-risk mothers this is even more important. My advice is to learn as much as you can about your disease process and how pregnancy affects your disease and you. Do not be afraid to bring new information to your physician or new details regarding your pregnancy. Both of you have a great investment in bringing forth a happy, healthy baby to join a wonderful loving family.

Epilogue

Well, we hope that your journey through this book has been and continues to be a memorable part of your pregnancy and childbirth experience. We have enjoyed sharing our experiences with you and thank you for the opportunity to do so. This wonderful book has truly been a labor of love. Our experiences will remain with us forever and be that much clearer because of this sharing.

If we have made you smile, laugh or reflect on the wonder of the life that your body is producing (or has produced) that makes this work we have put together all the more rewarding. Congratulations and much happiness to you and your beautiful baby. Be inspired and be encouraged, for you have witnessed a miracle. You have participated in the beauty of creation.

Appendix A
Internet Directory to
Pregnancy & Childbirth
Resources

If you frequent the internet and like to "surf the web (world wide web)," you might be interested to know that there is an overwhelming amount of information, as well as many fun sites, on pregnancy and childbirth. Even if you're a computer novice and you have access to the internet (through your home computer, a friend, your local library or cyber cafe), it might be worth it to check some of these sites out. Many of them are interactive aside from being informative.

Disclaimer: A listing here does not constitute an endorsement for any web site or server, nor does it speak to the accuracy of any of the information presented on these sites. This is strictly for informational purposes only. Similarly, exclusion from this listing does not say anything about a site. There are many fantastic sites not listed. The internet is changing and growing at about a million miles per hour. You'll have to find some of what you're looking for on your own. Keep in mind that the addresses we have provided are subject to change.

SPECIALTY SEARCH ENGINES:

🖰   **http://www.femina.com**

This site allows you to search topics related to women and has a "family and motherhood" search category which includes pregnancy and childbirth.

🖰   **http://www.wwwomen.com**

This site also allows you to search for topics related to women.

GENERAL SITES:

🖰   **http://www.babycenter.com**

A very comprehensive site with lots of good information. The site has various information areas including *pregnancy*, *preconception*, *dads*, *glossary*, *getting personal*, and a *baby monitor* area with the latest news and views.

The babycenter site is also customizeable (Check out sites with this feature if your're not familiar. You can make a custom page for the site that is your own entrance and guide). There are feature articles, shopping areas, chat areas and an *ask the experts* area.

The *ask the experts* area of this site includes as experts:

❀ 2 lactation consultants

❀ Dr. T. Berry Brazelton, a well known pediatrician

❀ 3 other pediatricians

❀ A male author of a book for dads

❀ 3 midwives

❀ A family practice physician

❀ A pediatric nurse practitioner

❀ 2 obstetricians

❀ A doula (a Greek word referring to a woman trained and experienced in childbirth and postpartum care)

🖰   **http://www.9months.com**

A site developed by a mother who was frustrated with the difficulty of buying maternity clothes and baby necessities. She seeks to make things easier for you!

⁐ **http://www.parentsoup.com**

Comprehensive site with a variety of offerings. You can "Join a pregnancy circle for the month you're due. Compare notes and share the joy with other parents-to-be."

Also features "specials" like a *baby name finder*, *book club*, *college calculator*, *virtual postcards*, etc. The various online communities include *expecting parent* and *parents of babies*. *The doctor is in* allows online chat with a physician. Experts available for your questions include a pediatrician and baby expert, as well as breastfeeding experts, etc.

⁐ **http://www.babybag.com**

Another comprehensive site that calls itself, "The In-Site to Parenting...Prenatal to Preschool."

It features numerous departments and interactive options, like bulletin boards (many different choices for diverse interests), birth announcement submission, book reviews, and *ask the professional*. On this site the professionals are:

❀ A pharmacist

❀ A childbirth educator

❀ A midwife

❀ a home based employment specialist

⁐ **http://www.storknet.org**

This is a pregnancy and parenting site. Some of the features include a *Father's Journal* column and a breastfeeding resource called *Breastfeeding Cubby!* You can also find shopping, pregnancy and parenting journals, and more.

⁐ **http://www.pregnancytoday.com**

This site is dedicated strictly to expectant parents. Among the areas to visit are a *Book Nook*, message boards, a due date calculator, birth stories, a *pregnancy daily* (customizeable page for every day of your pregnancy) and expert advice.

The experts on this site include:

❀ Nurse-midwives

❀ OB's

❀ Fertility specialists

❀ A lactation consultant

❀ Doulas

❀ A prenatal fitness instructor

❀ A childbirth educator

❀ A massage therapist

❀ A nutritionist

❀ An anesthesiologist

❀ A chiropractor/yoga instructor

🖰 **http://www.parents.com**
Big site from *Parents Magazine*. The pregnancy section includes *your pregnancy journal*, *what to expect obstetrician finder*, *childbirth planner*, *baby names*, *ask the ob/gyn*, and *new parent survival guide*.

🖰 **http://www.babyzone.com**
This site includes a *So, you're pregnant* page with good information. You can also go shopping for books, baby gear and maternity clothes. If you like chat, they have it and also *free stuff*, which everybody likes.

🖰 **http://www.parentsplace.com**
Large site whose index includes *children's health*, *pregnancy/fertility*, *marriage/family*, *recipes*, etc. The pregnancy and birth center includes *ask the midwife* and a variety of subject areas.

🖰 **http://www.acnm.org**
Website of the American College of Nurse-Midwives. Site includes information on Certified Nurse-Midwife education, *Find a Nurse-Midwife*, a bookstore, articles and more.

🖰 **http://www.dona.org**
Doulas of North America homepage

🖰 **http://www.familyweb.com**
An informative site with a pregnancy area. Includes a prenatal and postnatal

care table of contents, that leads to a lot of information.

🖱   **http://www.lalecheleague.org**

Information on breastfeeding from La Leche International

🖱   **http://www.babyworld.com**

Good information and resources

🖱   **http://www.annacris.com**

Retail site for Maternity Wear, plus useful links to other sites

🖱   **http://www.mothertime.com**

Retail site with Maternity Wear, Giftbaskets and links to non-retail baby
sites. Home site for national chain of maternity stores.

🖱   **http://www.bygpub.com/natural/**

Natural pregnancy and childbirth site. Areas include *natural family planning*,
healthy pregnancy tips, *natural childbirth*, *breastfeeding*, *family bed*, *attachment
parenting*, *infant massage*, *natural living*, and *home schooling*.

🖱   **http://www.efn.org/~djz/birth/birthindex.html**

The Online Birth Center with information on pregnancy, midwifery, birth
and breastfeeding. A comprehensive site.

🖱   **http://www.bradleybirth.com**

The Bradley Method of Natural Childbirth

🖱   **http://www.lamaze-childbirth.com**

Lamaze International. Site includes forums, pregnancy tips, info. on
programs, articles, papers, etc.

Happy Surfing!

Appendix B
Prenatal Care & Nutrition

One of the first things newly expectant mothers should do is take care of themselves. As you go, baby goes. Pregnant women have increased requirements for some very important vitamins and minerals. Unfortunately, most women in today's modern societies don't satisfy these increased demands through their diet. Your prenatal care, along with exercise, good nutrition and a positive attitude, are the keys to a beautiful pregnancy experience.

When you learn that you are expecting, make sure to ask your obstetrician about a prescription for prenatal vitamins.

Prenatal Vitamins:

These supplements are given to pregnant women to increase nutritional uptake in conjunction with the increasing demands your body and baby will place upon you. Your physician will usually have a favorite prenatal vitamin or at least one that he or she is familiar with. They will write a prescription for you based upon this.

Two of the very important needs that your pregnant body will have are for **Iron** and **Folic Acid**. Iron is essential to many bodily functions, including a strong immune system and, because of the increased blood volume of a mother-to-be, helping to form red blood cells. Iron also plays a role producing energy for the body.

Folic acid plays very important roles in the body as well. The manufacture of genetic material is one of the critical areas that folic acid impacts. It also affects the development of the central nervous system and the production of red blood cells.

A good prenatal multivitamin contains both Iron and Folic acid, but sometimes your physician may find it necessary to place you on an iron supplement or folate tablets, to make sure that you are receiving the necessary amounts of iron and folic acid.

For those who would like to also play an active role in keeping their body well maintained through diet, good sources of iron include meats (especially organ meats), poultry, fish, and soy products. Folic acid is found in fruits, legumes, grains and cereals, and dark green leafy vegetables.

Some of the other vitamins that can be found in prenatal multivitamin supplements include:

Vitamin B complex vitamins, some of which include:
❀ Thiamine (also known as Vitamin B1) helps with the conversion of carbohydrates into energy for mom and baby, impacting brain development. It is also important for a number of other developmental reasons.
❀ Riboflavin (also known as Vitamin B12) serves a broad range of functions including bone, and muscle development.
❀ Vitamin B6 is very important to your baby's brain development and nervous system. It also has important metabolic functions.

Vitamin C is important in the development of the body's resistance to infection, as well building connective tissue, etc.

Vitamin D is essential to bone development, among other things.

Calcium is a mineral that has been popular for a long time because of its role in forming strong bones, teeth, etc.

There are a host of other vitamins and minerals that are important and contained within prenatal multivitamin supplements. Your obstetrician is your best resource in this area and can recommend the appropriate prenatal vitamin for you.

Prenatal exercise:

Being pregnant doesn't mean simply lounging around and indulging food cravings. The proper exercise is also important. See Chapter 8, "Staying Fit," of this book.

Don'ts:

Especially in the 1st trimester, but throughout pregnancy, there are certain things that a pregnant woman should keep away from. As a general rule, alcohol, smoking, caffeine, uncooked seafood, and uncooked poultry or other meat products, should be avoided.

Another very important rule of thumb is that the mother-to-be should not take any medication without having discussed it with her doctor. Medications that you take can affect your baby.

Don't take the phrase, "You're eating for two now," literally. While your body's demands increase, it doesn't give mom an excuse to overdo it, especially with unhealthy concoctions of junk food.

Do's:

Enjoy your pregnancy!

Index

(where index references appear
for the names of the authors,
Elisa, Lorinda, Michelle and
Zaakira, page numbers mark
the beginning of a section of
commentary attributable to
that author)

A

abnormal fetal presen-
   tation 156, 194
   brow presentation
      195
   complete breech
      194
   face presentation
      195
   footling 195
   frank breech
      194, 195
abruptio placenta
   61, 156, 192, 213
active labor 139, 140
   contractions during
      140
   duration of 140
aerobic class 103, 108
aerobics 105
AFP. *See Alpha-
   fetoprotein*
alcohol 227
Alpha-fetoprotein 61
alternative childbirth
   methods 150
amenorrhea *61*
amnihook 153
amniocentesis *62*

amniotic fluid
   71, 146, 210
amniotic fluid embolism
   194
amniotic sac
   21, 153, 193
amniotomy 62, 153
anemia 190
   folic acid deficiency
      190
   iron deficiency 190
   sickle cell 190
anesthesia 141
ankle swelling 23
anti-hypertensive
   medications 203
anxieties 85
apgar scores 62
areola 62
   breastfeeding 62

B

baby 6
baby register
   items on 74, 75
baby registry 78
baby shower
   67, 69, 72, 73, 78
   baby registry 73
   when to have one
      67
baby showers 64
baby supplies
   67, 68, 69, 72, 74,
   75, 76
   Preparing Your Baby's
   New Home 76, 77
baby's development 21,
   52
   vitamins and minerals
      226
back labor 89
backache 23, 140

belching
   reasons for during
      pregnancy 45
belly button 23
belly wedge 23, 62
bikini incision. *See Low
   Transverse Incision*
birth 5, 148
   miracle xi
birth defects 202, 203
bleeding
   22, 137, 185, 186,
   191, 193, 207, 211,
   212, 213
   bright red blood
      22, 190, 192
   heavy bleeding 22
   causes 212
   light bleeding 191
bleeding gums 22
blood glucose 201
bloody show 136
body changes 82
body changes during
   pregnancy 43, 45
bonding
   7, 85, 86, 164
books 6, 13, 14
Bradley Method of
   Natural Childbirth
      223
brain hemorrhage 205
Braxton-Hicks contrac-
   tions
   23, 62, 136, 208
breast milk. *See
   mother's milk*
breast pump
   70, 162, 165
breast swelling
   27, 43, 46

breastfeeding
20, 161, 162, 163,
164, 166, 167,
170, 171, 174,
223
after c-section 158
baby latching on
162
bonding during
162, 164
effect on appetite
174
how long? 173
Breastfeeding Basics
171
breasts 104
breathing exercises
140
breathing techniques
150
breathlessness 22, 46
breech presentation
62, *194*
bright red blood *22*

C

c-section
36, 38, 39, 70, 89,
129, 131, 141,
155, 158, 192,
194
breastfeeding after
158
incision types 158
indications for 156
abnormal fetal
presentation 156
abruptio placenta
156
active maternal
herpes 156

cephalopelvic
disproportion
156
failure to progress
156
fetal distress 156
kidney disease
156
maternal diabetes
156
maternal hyper-
tension 156
overdue 156
placenta previa
156
prolapsed umbilical
cord 156
Low Transverse
Incision 71
pain after 164
pain following 157
urinary catheter
during 158
caffeine 21, 227
calcium 21, 205, 227
calcium channel
blockers 209
cardiovascular changes
during pregnancy
45
career
16, 95, 96, 98, 99,
100
cephalopelvic dispropor-
tion 156
Certified Nurse
Midwives 152
cervical evaluation 208
cervical polyp 212
cervix
26, 27, 70, 87, 132,
134, 138, 150,
153, 206

dilatation during
active labor 140
dilatation during
early labor 138
dilatation during
transition 142
cesarean section
155. *See also*
c-section
childbirth
6, 8, 14, 16, 30, 120,
121, 133, 143
delivery of the
placenta 147
final stage 147
importance of
support during 33
miracle
birth i, ii
Childbirth Preparation
Class 88, 120,
170
childcare 100
childcare leave 96
choriocarcinoma 193
chronic headaches 204
chronic hypertension
203
chronic lung disease
205
colostrum
70, 165, 166, 168,
169, 170, 171
role in elimination of
meconium 70
complications
189, 200
abnormal fetal
presentation 194
abruptio placenta
192
amniotic fluid
embolism 194
anemias 190

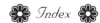

eclampsia 192
ectopic pregnancy
    191
fetal distress 196
gestational diabetes
    192
hyperemesis
    gravidarum 191
hypertonic uterine
    dysfunction 193
hypotonic uterine
    dysfunction 193
miscarriage 189
placenta previa 191
preeclampsia 192
premature labor 193
premature rupture of
    membranes 193
Rh incompatibility
    191
shoulder dystocia
    196
trophoblastic disease
    193
umbilical cord
    prolapse 194
urticaria 192
uterine hemorrhage
    postpartum 196
complications 205
conception 24, 52
confusion 22
congestion 46
constipation 21, 41
    prune juice 15
    reasons for during
        pregnancy 45
contractions 6, 14,
    62, 89, 90, 123, 137,
    138, 151, 208,
    213
    breathing during 89
    during transition
        142

irregular 136, 193
length of during
    active labor 140
length of during
    delivery 143
length of during
    early labor 138
length of during
    transition 142
monitoring 140
corticosteroid cream
    for urticaria 193
counterpressure 150
cravings 25. *See food
    cravings*
crowning 143, 150

D

D and C 190
delivery
    5, 9, 70, 132, 137,
    143
    duration of 143
delivery of the placenta
    147
Demerol 150
depression. *See
    postpartum blues*
diabetes 156, 201
    gestational 201
    pregestational
        and early
        miscarriage 202
    insulin dependent
        diabetes mellitus
        (IDDM/Type 2)
        201
    non-insulin
        dependent diabetes
        mellitus(NIDDM/
        Type 1) 201
diapers 76
diarrhea 207

digestive system
    changes during
        pregnancy 45
digital examination
    208
dilatation
    132, 138, 142, 193
dilation 70
doppler monitors 56
doula 220, 222
Down Syndrome 184
drinking *21*
due date 21

E

early labor 134, 138
    anxiety during 138
    dilatation during
        138
early pregnancy
    signs and symptoms
        27
eclampsia
    70, 192, 203
ectopic pregnancy
    70, 191
    signs and symptoms
        191
EDD. *See due date*
effacement
    70, 134, 138, 193,
    208
egg 26, 87
eighth month 23
Elisa
    6, 10, 14, 16, 20, 29,
    33, 37, 40, 42, 44,
    52, 53, 56, 64, 98,
    103, 124, 127, 148,
    155, 163, 167, 170,
    177, 186
embryo 27

emergency c-section
89, 156
in cases of abnormal
fetal presentation
195
emotions
16, 19, 42, 82
endocervical mucosa
212
engagement 134
engorgement
70, 162, 164, 171,
179
home remedies 162
epidural
129, 141, 149, 158
estimated due date.
See due date
estriol 208
estrogen
breast swelling 46
nipple tenderness 46
exercise
103, 105, 106, 108,
225
during pregnancy
105, 110
second and third
trimesters 109
expressing milk 165,
173

F

fallopian tube 191
fallopian tubes 26
false labor 62, 136
Family Leave of
Absence 92
fathers (expectant)
78, 79, 81
baby shower 86
Family Leave of
Absence 92

labor & delivery 83,
88
prenatal visits
84, 86
selecting obstetrician
84
fatigue 21, 82
fertilization 24
fetal birth defects 201
fetal distress 156, 196
fetal fibronectin 208
fetal heartbeat
27, 52, 56, 57
at 12 weeks 52
fetal lungs
constriction of
development 210
*See also pulmonary
hypoplasia*
fetal monitor 196
external 140
fetal monitoring
with epidural block
141
fetal movement
22, 23, 41, 53, 214
16 to 20 weeks into
pregnancy 54
in response to
stimulation 54
the sensation of
53, 54
time of day 54
fetal organs 199
fibroids 32, 41
fifth month 22
finances
95, 96, 97, 98, 100
first trimester 21, 227
flatulence 21, 23
Folic acid 225, 226
folic acid deficiency
190

food cravings 21,
27, 41, 42
foot growth during
pregnancy 44
forgetfulness 22
fourth month 22
frozen milk 163

G

Genesis 9
gestational age 205
gestational diabetes
192
gestational hypertension
203
God 5, 7, *29*
Goody Bag 123, 124,
140

H

hair growth during
pregnancy 43, 44
facial 44
heartburn
reasons for during
pregnancy 45
heavy bleeding 22
HELLP syndrome
192
hemolysis 192
high blood pressure
201.
See preeclampsia
high-risk pregnancy
148, 152, 199
defined 200
home pregnancy test
7, 20, 24, 25, 27, 28,
29, 34
Homebirth 151

hormonal changes
22, 46, 82
hormones 146
skin pigmentation
changes during
pregnancy 46
hospital bag
121, 122, 123, 124,
125, 127
hospital stay
private room 91
hospital tour 120
hyperemesis
gravidarum 191
hypertension 213
hypertonic uterine
dysfunction 193
hypotonic uterine
dysfunction 193

I

immune system 161
in-utero 10
incompetent cervix
207
incomplete abortion
190
indigestion 23
Indomethacin 209
induced labor
71, 87, 129, 137, 153
infertility 31
insomnia 23
insulin 192, 201
insulin resistance 192
insurance
notification of
company after
birth 91
internet 219
intrauterine growth
restriction
(IUGR) 203

intrauterine infection
211
Iron 21, 225, 226
Iron deficiency 22,
190

J

joint laxity 108

K

Kegel exercise 71
kidney disease 156

L

La Leche International
165, 171, 223
labor
i, 62, 120, 121, 132,
137, 138, 153,
170
phases of 137
labor and delivery
23, 85, 88, 89,
120, 150, 132,
133, 151
labor and delivery
room 88
lactation 71
lactation consultant
163, 165, 171
Lamaze International
150, 223
lanugo 146
laparoscope 191
Leboyer 151
leg cramps 23
let-down 71, *171*
lightening 71, 134
linea nigra 43

Lorinda 9, 13, 24,
30,38, 40, 41, 52,
53, 57, 72, 96,
122, 128, 148,
157, 164, 165,
170, 178, 186
Low Transverse
Incision 71
low transverse incision
159
lower esophageal
sphincter
changes in during
pregnancy 45

M

macrosomic growth
202
magnesium sulfate
209
marriage 30
maternal herpes 156
maternal hypertension
156
maternity care 152
meconium 71, 166
medication 21, 150
during labor
140, 141
membranes 71, 153
menstrual bleeding 31
menstrual cycle 26, 61
metastic trophoblastic
disease 193
methotrexate 191
Michelle
8, 14, 24, 30, 35,
40, 43, 51, 54,
57, 63, 96, 127,
131, 148, 157,
162, 169, 180,
184
midwife 71

midwifery 71, 152
midwives 151
miscarriage
30, 186, 201, 212
coping with 190
molar pregnancy 193
moles during pregnancy
43
mood swings
46, 82, 83
morning sickness 22,
25, 27, 41, 191. *See
also hyperemesis
gravidarum*
motherhood 9, 51
mother's milk 161
alcohol and drugs in
173
and diet 173
and prescription
medication 173
expressing 165
freezing and storage
163, 173
let-down 169, *171*
pumping 173
muscle conditioning
111
muscle toning 105
myomas. *See uterine
fibroids*

N

nail growth during
pregnancy 44
naps 82
nasal congestion 22
natural childbirth
149, 223
nausea 21, 27
incompetent cervix
213

New Parent Glossary
61, 62, 70, 71, 87, 90
newborn 171
appearance 146
color (pigmentation)
146
cup feeding 168
lanugo 146
pediatrician visit in
hospital 91
swollen genitals 146
nipple sensitivity 27
nipple tenderness 46
nipples 27
nosebleeds 22
nursery furniture
buying 65, 76
baby registry 74
themes 65
nursing
15, 64, 104, 162,
164, 171
nutrition 225

O

obstetrician 25, 38
finding 35, 37
importance of
34, 35, 37
oligohydramnios 210
onesies 66, 71
ovary 26, 191
ovulation 26, 28
Oxytocin. *See Pitocin*

P

parenting 8
pediatrician 62
contracting with 91
pelvic pain 31
perineal 87

phases of labor 137
Pitocin
71, 87, 129, 153, 193
placenta
26, 46, 87, 192,
193, 212
hormone production
46
placenta abruptio 203
placenta previa
87, 156, 191, 212
polyhdramnios 210
postpartum blues 87
postpartum paperwork
91
pre-milk. *See colostrum*
preconceptual counsel-
ing 200
preeclampsia
70, 87, 192, 203, 204
abdominal pain 204
chronic headaches
204
severe
HELLP syndrome
192
visual changes 204
Pregnancy Workout
Tips 107, 108
prelabor 134, 136
premature labor
193, 206, 208, 213
possible complica-
tions of 205
risk factors 207
treatment 209
warning signs 207
premature rupture of
membranes 193
premature rupture of
membranes 205
causes 210
complications 210

prenatal care
21, 31, 225
prenatal exercise
103, 106, 227
safety 110
prenatal visit 21
prenatal vitamins
21, 225
prepregnancy planning
200
preterm labor. *See*
premature labor
progesterone 22, 26,
46, 185
as cause of congestion
46
role in constipation
46
effects on lung
function during
pregnancy 46
effects on uterine
lining 46
prolapsed umbilical
cord 156
prostaglandin gel 153
Proverbs 22:6 8
prune juice. *See*
constipation
pulmonary hypoplasia
210
pushing
137, 142, 150
during delivery 143
urge to push during
transition 142
with epidural block
141
with spinal anesthesia
141

R

regional anesthesia 141

respiratory system
changes during
pregnancy 46
rest 15
Rh incompatibility
191
riboflavin 226
rooting 87, 171
rupture of membranes
62, 71, 137, 153, 193
delivery after 71
rupturing of membranes
infection 137

S

Sal Test 208
sciatic nerve 87
sciatica 87, 107
second pregnancy 20
second trimester 22
self-esteem 10
seventh month 23
shaking 149
shoulder dystocia 196
sickle-cell anemia 190
in pregnancy 191
sixth month 22
skin pigmentation
changes during
pregnancy 43
sleep deprivation 177
sleepiness 21
smoking 21, 227
as possible cause of
abruptio placenta
213
sodium 106
sonogram
35, 51, 52, 87
sonographer 35, 52
spinal anesthesia 141
spontaneous abortion
190

Spotting 90
spotting 185, 190,
191, 212, 213. *See*
also bleeding.
stages of labor 90
Stillbirth 190
stretch marks 44
stretching 107, 111
stuffy nose 46
swelling 106, 204
home remedies 106

T

tender nipples 21
Terbutaline pump 209
thiamine 226
third trimester 23
tragedy xii, 6
transition
90, 142, 150
trophoblastic disease
193

U

ultrasound xi, 21,
23, 27, 35, 52,
87, 204
fetal development 52
fetal heartbeat 52
fetal movement 52
vaginal probe 52
umbilical cord
father cutting 91
umbilical cord prolapse
194
urinary tract infection
191
urination
21, 22, 27, 45

reason for increase
during pregnancy
45
urticaria 192
uterine fibroids 31
uterine hemorrhage
postpartum 196
uterine infection 191
uterus
21, 22, 23, 26, 27,
31, 45
benefit of
breastfeeding 162
thickening of the
lining during
pregnancy 46

V

Vaginal Birth After
Cesarean. *See
VBAC*
vaginal canal 26
vaginal delivery 155
vaginal discharge
22, 23
varicose veins 44
VBAC (Vaginal Birth
After Cesarean)
39, 90, 159
vernix caseosa 146
villi 193
vitamin B complex
vitamins 226
vitamin B1. *See
thiamine*
vitamin B12. *See
riboflavin*
vitamin B6 226
vitamin C 226
vitamin D 227
vomiting 21, 27, 193

W

water breaking. *See
rupture of
membranes*
weight gain
24, 25, 40, 41
pre-pregnancy shape
103, 104
weight loss 105
weight training
104, 106
What's In Your Bag?
123

Y

your baby in the womb
23

Z

Zaakira
8, 15, 28, 32,
39, 42, 43, 51,
56, 68, 97, 121,
132, 149, 164, 166,
174, 179, 183